THE ORGANIC GUIDE
TO COLLEGES AND UNIVERSITIES

THE
Organic Guide
TO
Colleges and Universities

by the staffs of
Environment Action Bulletin,
Organic Gardening and Farming
and
Fitness for Living

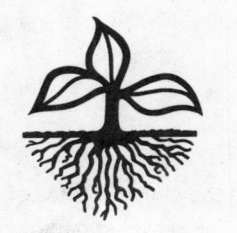

RODALE PRESS
Emmaus, Pennsylvania

The text for this book is based on
material which has appeared
in
ORGANIC GARDENING AND FARMING,
ENVIRONMENT ACTION BULLETIN
and
FITNESS FOR LIVING.

Printed in the United States of America
on recycled paper.

JB-2

First Printing—February, 1973

53499

CONTENTS

INTRODUCTION

It seems as if every day we learn of another course and another curriculum which should be included in this publication. We have tried to present the innovative work which has been done to teach students how they can live with an "environmental ethic" and how they can make a living from an environmentally-oriented job.

"Beginning this fall, 1972," writes biology professor Richard Null of Lane Community College in Eugene, Oregon, in a letter just received, "we plan to offer courses in organic gardening for which we will give college credit in Biology. We expect to have at least 90 students enrolled the first year. (Actually, more students are interested, but we must limit the enrollment the first year while we are getting the course going.) Our Board of Directors has authorized that the undeveloped grounds around the buildings, etc. be used by students and the community for their own garden plots."

Last week we learned that the Illinois Institute for Environmental Quality has sent 6,000 elementary school teachers in that state a copy of *Teaching Science with Garbage* as part of a classroom kit offering the best environmental education publications. Authored by Albert and Vivian Schatz and published by Rodale Press, *Teaching Science with Garbage* involves students in experiments showing how much garbage each produces at home, how it is handled by the community, and how it can be recycled by composting. Says Angela Emberman, the Institute's librarian, of the Environment in the Classroom packet: "We decided to do something about the problem of teachers having a hard time getting meaningful environmental education reference material and teaching aids."

Around the country, the need to solve problems in an environmentally-oriented way is developing job opportunities for trained personnel. Consider the use of pesticides. They're expensive pollutants. How do you farm without them? Thousands of farmers who are using organic growing methods are showing the way. But their results as well as their numbers would be increased if there were more Insect Ecologists—or whatever the descriptive term would be—advisers who would inspect fields on a regular basis and suggest cultural and biological controls as needed.

And trained people are needed in the marketing and merchandising of organically-grown and wholesome, natural foods. The American consumer wants more than agribusiness has been offering—and that should mean special training for people who will be making careers in that field.

Another area—this one in the engineering field—has to do with returning wastes to the land. As ocean dumping, burning and burying are recognized as uneconomical and unacceptable, it follows that trained people will be needed to develop alternatives. City public works departments will need agronomists, for example, as organic wastes from cities and industries are recycled into agriculture.

The United States Office of Environmental Education in Washington, D. C., is vitally interested in developing curricula in these areas. George Lowe of the office stresses the significance of an Integrated Pest Control curriculum which stresses cultural techniques and biological controls for insect pests. The curriculum, developed with the help of a grant from the Office of Environmental Education, is under the direction of Frank Bouwsma, Open College, Miami-Dade Junior College, Miami, Florida 33156. Mr. Bouwsma is the man who developed the "Man and Environment" general education course designed for either open-circuit or closed-circuit television.

A recent release from the Department of Health, Education and Welfare, noting that "not all educators and planners agree on a definition of environmental education, but they know what environmental education is and what it is not," defines the term as:

"A new approach to teaching about man's relationship to his environment—how he affects and is affected by the world around him;

"An integrated process dealing with man's natural and man-made surroundings;

"Experience-based learning, using the total human, natural, and physical resources of the school and surrounding community as an educational laboratory;

"An interdisciplinary approach that relates all subjects to a whole-earth 'oneness of purpose';

"Directed toward survival in an urban society;

"Life-centered and oriented toward community development;

"An approach for developing self-reliance in responsible, motivated members of society;

"A rational process to improve the quality of life;

"Geared toward developing behavior patterns that will endure throughout life."

"The consensus," it continues, "is that environmental education is not—

"Conservation, outdoor resource management, or nature study (although these may be included in an environmental education program);

"A cumbersome new program requiring vast outlays of capital and operating funds;

"A self-contained course to be added to the already overcrowded curriculum;

"Merely getting out of the classroom."

We hope this publication will stimulate further development of what we refer to as "organic" courses in the educational system. Hopefully, it will also serve to bring together people who share similar interests in environmental and organic education.

Jerome Goldstein
Editor, Environment Action Bulletin
August, 1972

CHAPTER I

THE ENVIRONMENTAL REVOLUTION IN NUTRITION EDUCATION

Robert Rodale

Suddenly, the teaching of healthful ways to eat is becoming of major interest to schools and colleges catering to students of all ages. Almost every day's mail brings to us reports of new, intensive and excitingly imaginative ways that nutrition and health are being taught to children, college students, and even adults. Often these courses combine nutrition education of the formal, technical kind with such closely related subjects as gardening and physical fitness—which give students important inspiration and added ways to put their nutrition knowledge to work.

The future looks even brighter. I predict that food and nutrition—and the whole idea of living naturally and organically—are soon going to become as basic as reading, writing and arithmetic in the curricula of schools. They will have to become that basic, in fact, if the human race is to stay strong, healthy and thriving, in the face of increasing inroads of "civilization diseases," with their fantastic cost for medical care. Every *school and college (and maybe even medical schools) will soon schedule food and nutrition studies as automatically as they now serve up traditional studies.* And people of all ages will sign up to take courses that will once and for all expose the mysteries of vitamins, minerals, enzymes, and nutrients of all kinds.

The beginning of the boom in nutrition studies—that we are seeing now—is a coming forth from the dark ages. Until recently, nutrition has been a suppressed subject, not only ignored but actually held down by forces of ignorance and repression. As a result, the average person in this country simply does not understand how to select a diet that will keep weight down, improve fitness and well-being, and assure health into the retirement years. Too many people have been putty in the hands of food companies that are overwhelmingly interested in profits, and only marginally mindful of nutrition.

All that is changing, though. We can now see ahead to the promised land, where people know enough about food to select a diet that is truly beneficial. I am sure that there will soon be a nutritionally educated segment of the population that will be a powerful force for improvement of food offered for sale, because they will know how to select what is good based on a true understanding of nutritional principles.

To understand why Americans are about to escape from nutrition ignorance, you should know how we got there in the first place. Here are the main reasons, as I see them:

1. For political and "national pride" reasons, we were for many years fed the shallow concept that "America is the best-fed nation on earth." The trappings of affluence and bulging supermarkets were confused with true nutritional adequacy. People were overfed but undernourished, and only the so-called food faddists realized that.

2. Nutrition teachers were for a long time the captives of the food industry. (Unfortunately many still are, but the number of independent teachers is growing rapidly.) The big money in food is made by processing and manipulating it, which also usually reduces its nutritional value. Those profits were used in subtle ways to capture the loyalties of home economists, nutritionists, and health educators whose minds were closed to any but the food industry party line on nutrition. While the nation's nutritional standard was going down, the nutrition profession was going down with it.

3. Criticism of bad food was brushed off effectively as "faddism." Much of the energy of nutrition teachers was devoted to cracking down on their critics, who they called quacks, distracting the public's attention from their own brand of false teaching.

Wrong education and bad nutrition leadership wasn't the only reason why national eating habits sank so low. Pockets of poverty caused some people to suffer from borderline starvation. And the sheer technological power of man to manipulate food brought us too far away from natural goodness, without any compensating philosophy of eating that could be understood by the mass of people.

We were truly in a wilderness, but those days are ending. Why? Because of the ecology movement, mainly. Suddenly people woke up to the almost deadly worsening of environmental quality. First, the air and water claimed most attention. Then people began to realize that food was the greatest environmental exposure of all, that there is an ecology of the body as well as of the biosphere. And environmental scientists helped too by looking for—and finding—pollutants in foods. Worries about pesticides, mercury, and depleted nutrients were on everyone's mind.

The revolution in nutrition education that I am talking about has itself been spawned by the ecology movement, in a very direct way. The teaching of ecology is now almost mandatory in all schools, even kindergartens. What used to be nature study is now environmental education, and what better way to teach people about the environment than to discuss their own personal ecology, using food as an example? By that route, the study of nutrition is being taken from the exclusive hands of the old-line home economists and is being packaged and sold by teachers who are exactly in tune with people's concerns of the day.

How beautiful a strategic maneuver that was! The old-line home economist, stirring her pot of Jell-O and handing out General Foods recipe leaflets, is bypassed. Pounding ahead like General Patton in a Sherman tank is the new breed ecologist who knows science well and bones up on enough nutrition (which is really not that complicated a subject, on the knife and fork level) to be able to teach accurately and effectively. It is like opening a door to a whole new world. Instead of being a drudge, nutrition is now an "in" subject.

I will tell you about one of the best of this new breed of teacher. He is Walter Tulecke, a botanist at the Science Institute of Antioch College in Ohio, an institution long known for innovation and inspired programs. Reacting to a letter to the editor in the school paper 3 years ago requesting a seminar in nutrition, Prof. Tulecke worked out an undergraduate general education course in nutrition. He expected 10 or 15 students to show up, but 120 came to the first meeting.

Breaking out of the traditional bounds of nutrition education, leaving the biases and strictures behind, he planned a course with many innovations. Lectures were given only twice a week. Many outside speakers were brought in. Movies were used, and field trips were held often. Students went to hospitals, a brewery, an organic farm, and held some of their discussion sessions in super-markets. They learned to prepare a dietary intake chart for a day, weighing all their food and determining its nutritional value.

"One of the unusual aspects of this course is the serving of food in class," Tulecke says. That sounds like it would be routine for the study of the science of food, but you can't imagine how restrictive some concepts of food teaching have been. A clue to the tone of the class is revealed by the listing of foods Walter Tulecke says have been served: homemade cottage cheese, peanut bread, garbanzo patties, high protein muffins, survival food for backpacking, soybean casserole, supercheap foods, kasha, yogurt, and so forth. A vegetarian restaurant was started by one group of students, and a good food co-op by others. The co-op now has 800 members, including many non-students from neighboring towns.

There is a garden in this picture too, as at the Santa Cruz campus of the University of California. "A quarter of an acre of golf course turf was turned under, fertilized with manure, campus leaves and compost, and planted to vegetables of many different types," Tulecke says. That organic garden, also worked by townspeople, became a focal point of the nutrition studies.

"The garden," says Tulecke, "was a good place for discussions and it frequently became a small learning center related to nutrition, soils, biological control and many other subjects."

The most important thing about a class like this—a feeling which is hard to put into words—is the sheer *freedom* of learning a subject like nutrition when it is taught in the new atmosphere of openness. Released from the need to follow the party line of the food processors, a teacher of nutrition can make the subject exciting and involving. Under the old system, nutrition teachers were afraid to get their students too excited about the subject for fear they would turn into faddists. That's true! Caring too much about food, becoming passionate about its health values, is a sign of pathology to a traditional nutritionist.

The new wave rolls on, though, over the heads of the oldtimers. Walter Tulecke is just one of the new breed. Even more radical, yet with perhaps more pertinent academic orientation, is health teacher Norma C. Westcott. Her new type of health and nutrition program is called "Prescription for Life," and her students are 310 eighth graders of the Shendehowa Central School District near Albany, New York.

"Public health experts have just about given up on the current generation of adults," the N. Y. *Times* says in reporting on the program. One of her goals is to train young people to be general health counselors—to teach preventive medicine concepts to their friends and even to their parents.

In fact, these kids can be pretty hard on their parents. "My mother is killing me," one student reported to his class. How? By making him eat a breakfast with too much fat. Mrs. Westcott's students learn more than nutrition, though. They know how to take each other's pulse, blood pressure, and can even work electrocardiogram machines. After exercising regularly, they see how their hearts become trained, and how their bodies can do more work with less strain on their cardiovascular systems.

The idea of making eighth graders into health counselors is fascinating, to say the least. It is a practical idea too, and a great example of the kind of nutritional and health-education advances that can be made once people start looking beyond the facade of prestige and degrees that has entangled the health-care professions. Many people are now thinking along that route, not just Mrs. Westcott. The President's Council on Health Education, spoke out on the same issues. The committee staff indicated to me that it is distressed with the parochialism and petrified career structure of the health professions, and that new ways must be found to teach people rapidly to help others to better health.

Don't think that all this will happen only to other people. You can be a part of this new movement toward a nutrition and health awakening. You must be interested, or you wouldn't be reading this book. And it is interested people who are going to keep this growing idea of real nutrition education moving along.

CHAPTER II

BECOMING A PERSONAL HEALTH EDUCATOR

John Haberern

On first thought, the idea that you can begin to teach others about fitness and health may seem a bit far out to you. Perhaps even a bit daring.

In this day and age of mounting degenerative diseases, soaring medical costs and a health care system built around the "breakdown-patch up" philosophy, it becomes increasingly obvious that preventing rather than curing disease is the only hope of the future.

In his book *University at the Crossroads* the medical profession's distinguished historian H. E. Sigerist, points up the problem with a quotation from Sir George Newman: "The ideal of medicine is the prevention of disease, and the necessity for curative treatment is a tacit admission of its failure."

Unfortunately, under present conditions, the concept of preventing disease is foreign to the practice of most physicians. Says Edward J. Steiglitz, M.D., in *Time* magazine, "The trouble is that doctors think entirely in terms of disease, and are ignoring their opportunities for making people healthier." The medical profession will argue that it has taken great strides in disease prevention by educating people to be vaccinated or immunized, to have a chest x-ray, to use seat belts, and with certain symptoms to avoid delay in seeing a physician. Those activities do produce results. Death and disabilities are being prevented through educational activities related to the early detection of cancer, heart disease, tuberculosis, glaucoma and other health problems.

But again, this type of thinking and activity is entirely disease oriented. Up to this point, little if anything has been done by physicians to help make people healthier. The answer, says H. E. Sigerist in *University at the Crossroads*, lies in cultivating an entirely new attitude in the medical profession. "The student must be interested in health, not only in disease."

Of course, it would be unfair to place all the blame for our nation's deplorable health at the feet of physicians. Physicians are so busy patching up and treating conditions which are the result of our lifelong insane living habits that they have very little time to devote to health education. Anyway, says Roger J. Williams, Ph.D., professor of biochemistry at the University of Texas, "Under present conditions they are paid for bringing their patients back to health; they are not paid when the patients stay healthy. Although that sounds merciless and unhumanistic, it is a fact of life. "This is a real problem which the medical profession will somehow have to solve" Dr. Williams writes in the May-June, 1972, issue of *Nutrition Today*, "We need able physicians, and they need to be paid well; but we must find someway to avoid this 'breakdown-patch up' philosophy."

No, I don't think we can look to physicians as a group to provide the setting and stimulation for people to change old health practices or to adopt new ones. Undoubtedly, some physicians take the time to counsel their patients on health matters and others serve as advisors or resource people for community health education programs. At best, such services reach only a handful of the population and usually involves only those people who make the initial contact because of some illness or disease. It is unusual for the person who is supposedly "healthy" to go to a physician for services other than health check-ups and disease screening tests. How many people do you know who consult their doctor about things they can do to improve their fitness and health?

It is unrealistic, too, to think that the present methods of consumer health education are going to get the job done. Dr. Scott K. Simonds, Professor of Health Education at the University of Michigan School of Public Health, told the August 1971 American Health Congress, "It is not enough to pass out pamphlets in waiting rooms, or set up exhibits in the corridors of hospitals. It will not be sufficient to run a television program every so often."

President Nixon in his Health Message to the 92nd Congress made the same point. "We have given remarkably little attention to the health education of our people. Most of our current efforts in this area are fragmented and haphazard. A public advertisement once a week, a newspaper article once another week, a short lecture now and then. There is no national instrument, no central force, to stimulate and coordinate a comprehensive education program," the President emphasized.

What we need to remedy this situation, according to Dr. Simonds, is "active consumer participation in the health system." And to do that there has to be personal contact, people working with others on a one-to-one basis or in small groups. As Bob Rodale points out, "It is possible for people who have not been trained formally in physical education, health or education to be leaders, teachers and advisors. We have known of many such people, who have a deep interest in trying to know more about health, and who have become very effective leaders. Many times such people, who have taught themselves the basic facts of physiology, nutrition and health, are far more effective teachers than those who are formally trained, because they communicate with people on their own level, not as experts."

ONE PROGRAM TO DEVELOP PERSONAL HEALTH EDUCATORS

YMCA-FITNESS FINDERS is a series of classes, held once a week, that teach people about health and especially about exercise. Y-FITNESS FINDERS is more like a club than a class. Men, women, and sometimes whole families get together for an hour in the evening—sometimes during the day. They wear comfortable clothes and bring along the desire to pare a few inches from hips or waist, learn how to strengthen hearts and lungs. There's a little bit of talking at a YMCA-FITNESS FINDERS session, and a lot of mild, rhythmic exercises done to catchy music.

People quickly unbend at FITNESS FINDERS. The accent is on informality, fun, learning, and movement. You walk around in a circle to warm-up, pumping your arms to loosen up shoulder muscles. Then you jog a little, and even kick your heels if you want to. You bend and stretch, and learn special exercises to relax, or to get your body in shape again.

FITNESS FINDERS was created by Rodale Press several years ago to meet the need for a way to motivate people to exercise safely and to learn about health. Our purpose in planning FITNESS FINDERS was to work out a series of classes that would combine health lectures with physical movement in a format of fun and group dynamics. Spreading this scientifically correct and popular program across the country was a tremendous challenge, though. We needed many qualified fitness instructors with the right personality and training. Finding them was difficult.

Then it hit us. The YMCA's have the trained physical educators, so why not approach them about introducing people across the country to FITNESS FINDERS? We did, and Y-FITNESS FINDERS was born. Today there are more than 1,200 instructors running classes in over 200 locations.

Even more important is the fact that Y-FITNESS FINDERS is only the first in a series of Y programs designed to help people who are interested in finding health naturally. The YMCA-FITNESS FINDERS school program was the next step.

In the Y-FF system, health and physical education is taught as an integrated unit in the same course.

Health education has to shift gears. No longer do we have to give as much emphasis to girding children for the battle against infectious diseases. In the nineteenth century before sanitation and infectious disease were brought under control by sanitary knowledge and antibiotics, infectious disease was the great killer of mankind. The bad, killer diseases of today, however, don't come into our systems from dirty water or insect bites. They "infect" us in our clean homes often because we are following self-indulgent patterns of living which prevent our bodies from reaching and maintaining an adequate level of fitness. The seeds of some of these degenerative diseases are planted in youth, or even in childhood, and they get a foothold in our bodies years before their presence is revealed either by symptoms or results of medical tests or examinations. According to Dr. Leona Baumgartner, former Commissioner of Health in New York City, "In the middle of the twentieth century, we are dealing with a host of chronic diseases including cancer and atherosclerosis, ailments that may be prevented by what people do by themselves in the way of eating, smoking and exercise."

YMCA-FITNESS FINDERS for schools is doing exactly what Dr. Baumgartner and other forward-looking health and exercise researchers recommend as a way out of our modern degenerative disease dilemma. Children are getting the education, guidance and inspiration they need to help themselves develop the habits that will build resistance to modern health problems.

A special pilot Y-FITNESS FINDERS program for 5 fifth and sixth grades in the San Diego City School System began in January, 1973.

"In the past," says National FITNESS FINDERS Director Charles Kuntzleman, "health education and physical education were two distinct parts of the school curriculum. Health was concerned primarily with concepts, understandings and attitudes about living effectively in order to reduce disease and improve personal and community health practices. Physical education, on the other hand, was concerned with body activity designed to develop physical resources in order to provide stamina, strength, and efficient movement for full and complete living."

What we've done is integrate health education and physical education. Take the unit on the circulatory system, for example. Here the emphasis is on how the child's total living pattern—his life style—influences his heart, blood vessels and blood. Basic to the whole program is daily or alternate day physical activity. And since health and physical education are integrated, the physical activity in this unit is geared toward activities designed to improve the circulatory system. Such things as relays, rope skipping, aerobic games and other endurance-producing exercises.

As part of the same class session, the students use manuals and workbooks to learn how they can keep tabs on their circulatory system by monitoring such things as pulse rate and blood pressure. They also learn how to keep their heart and vascular system in tip-top shape by selecting low cholesterol diets, and foods low in white sugar and white flour. In addition, they learn why it is important to get the right kind and amount of cardiovascular exercise, how smoking and drugs play havoc with their bodies and why air pollution hinders the heart's ability to pump blood through the thousands of miles of blood vessels.

Using the workbooks as a guide, the students take their own pulse rates and blood pressures and soon discover how physical activity, certain foods, smoking, age, and sex differences affect their circulatory system. The San Diego children will also be taking the pulse rates of their parents and explaining why there is a difference between their heart rate and that of their parents. They will be taking the pulse rates of smokers and non-smokers and explaining why there is a difference.

"In this small way," Charles Kuntzleman explains, "children can actually be health counselors for their parents. When a child can explain to his father what a jump of 20 beats or more in pulse rate after smoking only one cigarette means in terms of his heart health and his chances eventually of avoiding coronary, there is a good chance that that father may be adding years to his life by cutting down on smoking. That's real health education taking place."

In the "Getting Back to Nature" unit, for instance, pupils study the relationships that exist between the various components of health and fitness in their own bodies. Then, building on this knowledge, they begin to explore the bonds by which man is linked to other living things.

For example, when a biological concept such as bilateral symmetry, or warm blooded animals vs. cold blooded animals, or the vertebrate body plan is introduced we illustrate the similarities and differences between the human body and the bodies of other vertebrates. When we talk about the life in the soil, the intention is to show the student how dependent he is on the soil, even if he rarely gets out of the city or suburbs.

Activities for each unit are designed to encourage the pupil to use his senses to *discover*, to ground his theoretical knowledge on a first-person acquaintance with the workings of nature. All of the instructional materials, as well as the manner in which they are to be presented, are aimed at heightening the child's sensitivity to his environment and helping him play a responsible role in its preservation.

In each unit, the reading assignment is supplemented by student projects and supportive learning activities, both

11

53499

indoor and outdoor. In the soil unit, for instance, the pupil works on projects that drive home the practical significance of organic matter in the soil, water erosion, soil micro-organisms, soil temperature and texture, etc. Instead of merely reading about how to take a soil profile, how to increase the soil's water absorption capacity, and how a compost pile works, the students learn by doing.

A premium is placed on practical knowledge—the kind of knowledge that provides access to an organic way of living. By the time he completes the "Back to Nature" unit, the student knows how to make and read maps, as well as how to find his way in the wilderness, with or without a compass. He will be able to estimate height, weight and length using only materials found in nature. He'll know how to make weather instruments, and how to forecast and record weather information. He will know how to attract birds to his backyard, how to forage for wild foods, how to tell a good bug from a bad bug, how to sprout seeds and grow a windowsill garden, how to read a food label, and how to tell the difference between organic and non-organic foods, and he will participate in dozens of other valuable learning activities never before offered in the traditional health and physical education program.

Another example of how Y-FITNESS FINDERS is moving in the direction of a total health education program is the recent Y-FF credit course at Clark Community College in Vancouver, Washington. "Clark decided in favor of the program due to the strength of the programs' educational materials, its format, and its 12-week cycle which fits into its quarter hour system," said Henry Fowler, executive director of the Vancouver YMCA. "It was also accepted strongly because the educational material was extensive enough to allow it to be extended from quarter to quarter for more advanced classes."

Added Fowler, "The real dynamics of this program as a credited college course lie in its capacity for teaching the requirements for personal fitness, gauging achievement through pulse rates, body measurements, etc. It's fun and fits into the physical activity requirements of any P.E. course. Another important factor was that it helped the participants develop outside fitness interests via the CV program."

CHAPTER III

ANN ARBOR: TEACHING A COMMUNITY TO GARDEN

Jerome Goldstein

In Ann Arbor, Michigan, pressure has surfaced into action in a variety of ways. The movement toward a more natural and meaningful life bubbles over into food cooperatives, community organic gardens, courses in the University of Michigan there, local environmental action groups and more.

The municipality is becoming involved. The citizens and students are becoming involved. The whole direction and tenor of life there is changing subtly as the citizens face the incredible fact that the dream of a life of ease and affluence was a greedy and selfish dream at best.

This is the story, most of it told by the prime movers involved, of the beginnings of that change, the re-establishment of community identity, the sharing and working together to handle life-support functions, and the force that is moving locally and powerfully in this country.

In January 1972, I was invited to give a talk at the University of Michigan on "Organic Force, Social Practice and Harmony with the Environment." It was part of a 1972 seminar series, "Man Adapting to the Small Planet."

While preparing the paper, I found myself always coming back to the same points:

• The organic idea is small, simple, warm and personal (like a compost pile), thus in sharp contrast to Big, Mass, Brand-Name Ideas all around us;

• Organic force can bring people back into the marketplace, and pay for them to be there (prime example: organic farming producing food that is eventually sold in mama-and-papa neighborhood stores in cities);

• The beauty of the organic idea as a social force is

that it is firmly rooted in materials, methods and efforts which most people usually refer to as garbage, idealistic, inefficient or economically unfeasible. (Organic force brings economy and ecology together, and shows how to make a profit without messing up the environment.)

To make the above points, I referred to the *Blueprint for Survival* developed by Edward Goldsmith and a team of British scientists; to Jane Jacobs, author of *The Economy of Cities;* and Wendell Berry, Kentucky poet-farmer-professor. The first two stressed that cities must start treating their garbage as resource and relate to agriculture if urban life is to be livable. I hoped these references and others made clear how organic force was surfacing in many different areas and could revolutionize society to the benefit of us all.

Then I got to Ann Arbor, and 12 hours later I realized that the organic force I had merely spoken about was already well under way there—it was alive and well thanks to the efforts of a small group of citizens.

At the center of that small group is Bill Kopper, an unassuming 23-year-old with a steady, even voice that seems perfect for bringing a variety of people together. Bill had been the first director of the Ann Arbor Ecology Center.

The center serves as a focal point for supplying environmental information and coordinating projects, ranging from a just-developing commodity exchange store, where citizens can swap products and services, to a highly organized recycling program that more than 25,000 people have participated in since it began. Says Pat Taylor of the center: "Since opening our new station, we are handling 16,000 pounds of glass, 2,500 pounds of cans, and 12,000 pounds of papers per day on a 4-day work week of 26 hours. We're now working with city officials to develop a plan to involve the city more directly."

Like most college communities, Ann Arbor has a great organic restaurant—Indian Summer—and it was filled with University of Michigan students when we got there for lunch. Although Indian Summer hadn't forced the nearby Gino's to close down, the possibility was discussed—unless Gino's goes organic first.

After lunch came a meeting with the Ann Arbor Organic Garden Committee—a truly remarkable bunch. In

January 1971, a group of Ann Arbor citizens, Washtenaw County farmers, and University of Michigan students and faculty met to plan a Community Organic Garden. "These people," Bill Kopper explains, "helped provide the political clout to persuade the Executive Committee of the University to provide a seven-acre lot for the Community Garden. The group also helped obtain an initial $5,000 grant from the university's Institute for Environmental Quality."

This year, the Organic Garden Committee has worked its way out of the garden and into the entire community. Its interests and technical expertise range from pesticide usage to nutrition. Decisions at the biweekly meetings go from the design of this year's Community Garden to ways of working with food co-ops and aiding a county nutrition program that emphasizes vegetable proteins.

One subject for discussion the day I sat in on the committee was how to extend the benefits of the People's Co-op (which now serves students) to the poorer neighborhoods of Ann Arbor. To work this out, representatives of the Office of Economic Opportunity and the Co-op attended the meeting. Early in its history, the Co-op decided to buy as much organic food as possible and to purchase primarily from small farmers. According to Bill Kopper, the People's Co-op has become an "organic force" over the past years because of the willingness of people to go to a little extra bother to obtain good quality food.

Susan Drake and John Strider are organizing the neighborhood garden project called GROW. The different sites are on land owned by the school system and the city as well as private people—one plot is 10 acres. The City Council has enthusiastically endorsed the garden project, as have the Chamber of Commerce, Consumers for Enact and the Ann Arbor Garden Club. All kinds of benefits are described by Mrs. Drake in a statement she issued on the neighborhood garden concept. "Garden activity draws together people of all social and economic backgrounds," she said. "Differences of age, race, income and political thought are bridged by the shared experience of working on a plot of ground." The object of the committee is to make gardening a basic activity available to all residents of Ann Arbor, and project GROW is well prepared to do just that!

The rain was turning to sleet as we drove out to the

15

North Campus and the seven-acre Community Organic Garden. Dr. Robert Zahner, professor in the School of Natural Resources (and prime mover), and John Remsberg, graduate student (and garden manager), have a well planned garden—having had the advice of about 60 students in John's three-credit course, "Living with the Earth."

Hundreds of people worked in the garden last year and shared in the harvest, which Bob Zahner says was tremendous. In the information sheet on the garden, much emphasis is given to the "public laboratory" quality which shows the effectiveness of different kinds of composting, mulches, companion plantings and biological control methods. But it's also more than a demonstration of scientific and chemical-free methods of yard and garden care, says Bob: "It strives to provide a complete educational experience which will involve people in the active process of change in life style, needed to insure a livable environment in the future."

If you look around wherever you live, chances are that there are more good things going on than you ever thought possible. That's the special quality of Organic Force—steady, quiet, local and most effective.

THE ANN ARBOR ORGANIC GARDEN COMMITTEE . . .

In January 1971, a group of Ann Arbor citizens, Washtenaw County farmers, and University of Michigan students and faculty met to plan a Community Organic Garden. As plans progressed, some people found that they didn't like to attend meetings and they dropped out of the group; but new people were quickly found to take their place. During April, the Garden Committee persuaded the Executive Committee of the University to provide a seven-acre lot for the Community Garden. The group also helped obtain an initial $5,000 grant from the Institute for Environmental Quality, and added credibility to a larger grant application to the Office of Education.

Today the Organic Garden Committee is serving a somewhat different purpose. It has become a community-wide repository of technical expertise on such topics as pesticide usage, nutrition, soil monitoring, horticulture and organic technique. In the meetings every other week, decisions are made about the design of the Community Garden, ways of working with good co-ops, and plans for a county nutrition program emphasizing vegetable proteins. Frequently, the discussions take a somewhat philosophical bend, and the committee members talk about where they would like to go with the different programs and how they might bring along the entire community.

Because of the diverse backgrounds of the people who have worked on the Organic Garden Committee, the committee has developed into a coordinating body for the many different groups involved with organic foods and organic growing.

. . . AND THE COMMUNITY ORGANIC GARDEN

The Community Organic Garden demonstrates to the residents of the Washtenaw County area that pesticides and chemical fertilizers are not necessary for urban lawn and garden care. In addition, the garden serves as a public laboratory to show the effectiveness of different kinds of composting, various mulches, companion plantings and methods of biological control of insects. However, the garden achieves more than the demonstration of scientific and chemical-free methods of yard and garden care. It strives to provide a complete educational experience.

In order to realize the goals of the garden, an educational committee made up of volunteers is promoting the following projects:

• Developing insect collections designed to serve as a teaching tool to help people identify pests and learn nonchemical control of insects.

• Scheduling visits to the garden by civic clubs, public school classes, church groups and other organizations.

• Publishing booklets describing different techniques of organic gardening and printing articles on the garden in newspapers in Washtenaw County.

• Building a library which will be of value to the community in the search for ecologically preferred solutions to lawn and garden problems.

• Collecting and laminating specimens of weeds and

wild plants to help the public learn how to control problem plants and to identify edible or poisonous plants.

• Presenting research in soil composition, the relationship between gardening methods and productivity, and the effectiveness of certain types of companion planting.

• Demonstrating recycling of garbage, glass, paper, sawdust, woodchips, wood ashes, manure and weeds.

• Providing the opportunity for social interaction between professors, students, farmers, veterans, retirees, Girl Scouts, and others in working and non-working situations.

Ann Arbor's Community Organic Garden is an experiment in education, and hopefully it will help define values which will correct the environmental inequities generated by a culture that does not understand what it is dependent upon.

(The preceding information was prepared by Project Community Education, 417 Detroit Street, Ann Arbor.)

GROW: A NEIGHBORHOOD GARDEN PROJECT

Susan Drake and John Strider

This proposal will make gardening a basic activity available to all residents of Ann Arbor. The potential for neighborhood gardens is tremendous.

There is most definitely a demand for a gardening program in Ann Arbor at this time. Over 400 people participated in the Community Organic Garden on the North Campus.

Individual efforts to establish community gardening were apparent in the past. At the corner of Stone School and Ellsworth Roads, 43 families got together and gardened on land made available by a private Ann Arbor firm. There was an unusual drought that suppressed plant growth but not the people's enthusiasm. Other efforts at neighborhood gardening were successful in the past and are being explored.

Two of the many sources of impetus behind a community-wide gardening program have been indicated above:

Efforts on the part of individuals and the Community Organic Garden with Ecology Center sponsorship. An informal organization called GROW is attempting to put all these forces into one cohesive framework. It is envisioned that numerous neighborhood-run gardens would be assisted concurrently by the Recreation Department, the Community Organic Garden/Ecology Center, the County Extension Service and all other interested community organizations. The following endorsements have been received: Advisory Committee to the Recreation Department, Ann Arbor Ecology Center/Community Organic Garden, and the Ann Arbor Garden Club. Encouragement has been offered by: The Chamber of Commerce, County Extension Service, Housing Commission, Ozone House and Public School System. Other organizations that will hopefully lend support include: Senior Citizens, Model Cities, Church youth services, Boy and Girl Scouts, 4-H, handicapped children's organizations, AAUW, and community service clubs such as Kiwanis, Optimists, and Jaycees. A resolution supporting the program was passed by the Ann Arbor City Council.

The following are the major goals of the neighborhood garden program:

(1) It is desired that the opportunity of gardening be made available to all Ann Arbor residents. A number of garden sites will increase the opportunities. Present commitments for land include: Northside Park/School, Ecology Center Recycling Depot, Pioneer II High School, Stone School-Ellsworth Road site. Numerous other sites are well suited to the program and permission for their use is being sought.

(2) Perhaps the most obvious result of a gardening program will be the supply of produce that people can raise. Relatively inexpensive, high-quality and nutritious vegetables are increasingly rare. The freshness of home grown produce is unsurpassed.

(3) A major objective of the overall program is to develop a sense of community. Providing a common neighborhood project such as a garden is a proven method of drawing people together to cooperatively work and learn from each other.

(4) Developing a greater community awareness of our environment is one fundamental concept of the garden program. There is no better way to "get back to the earth" than to work with the soil and plants and observe life on

that basic level. Such an experience puts current issues of land conservation, ecology and pollution into perspective.

(5) The garden program is intended to make a fundamentally unique contribution to the variety of life in Ann Arbor. By providing a gardening recreation program, an alternative that is now lacking and yet highly desired will be available. Viewed as focal points for activity, neighborhood garden sites offer a counterpoint to the usual urban environment.

(6) A primary goal of the program is to encourage youth participation. Along with the growing concern for the environment among young people is the fact that certain children are disenfranchised from ordinary urban youth programs. Disadvantaged and handicapped children especially could be involved with a neighborhood garden program.

(7) The senior citizens of the community have a tremendous amount of expertise in gardening, and this resource can be called on by a community garden project. Although some of these citizens may not be able to participate physically in a garden, they are willing to serve as advisers. If the garden program encourages the participation of this segment of the community, all of Ann Arbor will benefit.

To realize the goals outlined above, the following programs will be initiated:

(1) In providing the opportunity to garden, sites for this activity will be made available on public and private land. All people who wish to be involved may do so; the only limitation will be size. Family plots (30 x 50 feet) can be laid out and occupied on a first-come, first-served basis. If people desire to merge their plots, they may do so. Arrangement of plots within the site, what to grow and other matters will be left to the people at each location.

(2) Essential resources for gardening will be made available. These include water, plowing, some seed and plant materials, rock powders and organic matter, and tools on a lend-out basis. Information in the form of a biweekly newsletter and radio and newspaper coverage will inform people on how to garden as well as what to watch for on the plot. Some of these items may be offered as donations by members of the community. To encourage participation

of all people, a supply of basic resources must be available.

(3) The value of having a number of garden sites around the city is that it encourages participation on a neighborhood level. For the first year about ten pilot gardens were emphasized. The sites now committed and those that are being sought are distributed around the major areas of the town. Run by the people of each area, each garden will be a local cooperative project.

(4) The educational potential of the program is enormous. First, the primary contact of people with each other on a garden site will be very strong. Past experience verifies the strength of interaction between people while gardening. As part of the overall program, on-site discussions will be organized for all interested groups. To deal with topics such as gardening, ecology, biology and land conservation, local people with knowledge in these areas will be available to talk. An index of these people will be kept on file.

(5) As a regular element of summer activity, neighborhood gardens offer a diversity of possibilities. With few minor facilities, picnicking, relaxation, handicraft arts, painting and philosophy can all be engaged in at garden sites. Gardens are ideal for small, informal gatherings and family activities and will quickly become a unique activity point in the community.

(6) A variety of possibilities exist to encourage participation by young people. Handicapped and disadvantaged children, 4-H, Boy and Girl Scouts and Church youth groups can all plug into the program. In addition, summer job corps organizations can very easily be accommodated. Along with instruction on gardening, biology and ecology, the young people involved can assist in site preparations, construction of compost bins and picnic benches and helping to teach others.

(7) Acting through the Senior Citizens' Council, all people in that organization will be invited to participate. They will be invited to act as consultants as well, if they so desire. A file of people who agree to be so involved will be kept.

In order to implement such a wide-scale program it is necessary to have a basic staff and many committed volunteers.

A program coordinator is needed to coordinate the overall development of the various garden site activities. It is the coordinator's responsibility to assist each neighborhood in site and program development in response to its unique need and desires.

The coordinator will recruit and make available recreational and educational resource people and materials. It is his or her responsibility to work in conjunction with various agencies such as 4-H, the Community Organic Garden and the recreation department to make existing programs available at neighborhood garden sites and to develop new programs and resources.

The director will establish a manpower pool to be made available for specific and general projects at each site. Included in this pool will be persons with planning expertise and gardening experience, youth supervisors, and a corp of young adults to assist with the planning and actual building of the physical site and to assist in the planning and implementing of various on-site activities.

One aspect of establishing garden sites is to promote community involvement, and the director will be seeking new ways of accomplishing this. A great loss in many urban areas is the sense of neighborhood and group identity and participation. The director will establish and maintain communication with as many groups as possible and will try to provide specific and general activities involving the elderly, handicapped (we have seed funding for a program working with the handicapped), emotionally disturbed and other generally isolated individuals and groups.

Community involvement should extend to those individuals who may perhaps have something to give or share with a program. The coordinator will be seeking assistance from service organizations, the fire and police departments, churches and other existing groups.

CHAPTER IV

FOOD CONSPIRACIES

"The closer you get to the source of organic food, the cheaper and fresher the food will be and the better you'll feel about it."

William D. Kopper

On October 7, 1971, Washtenaw County Weights and Measures inspectors made simultaneous raids on three Kroger stores in Ann Arbor, Michigan. Their discovery shocked the community. In two of the three stores, over half the meat packages were underweight, and in the third store all the meat in the display case was underweight. The Broadway Kroger, where I was forced to do my shopping before joining the Co-op and which incidentally serves the poor section of town, was the store with 100 percent violations. Each package of meat was overpriced between five and twenty-five cents, bringing the store more than $200 per day illegitimate profit. However, the Kroger stores were not the only chains found cheating during the October raids in Ann Arbor; in nine of the fifteen other stores inspected, serious violations were detected. A few weeks later a similar series of investigations of chain store meat departments were conducted in that western part of the state. An appalling 70 percent were found to be short-weighing their meats.

Bob Harter, Washtenaw County Supervisor of Weights and Measures, decided to conduct the October raids in Ann Arbor after a methodical investigation indicated that most stores in the area were cheating the consumer. When questioned about the epidemic of short-weighing meats, he cited inspections in other parts of the state and throughout the country as evidence that is is probably a nation-wide trend. Although Kroger probably did not send a policy memo to its stores telling them to under-weigh their meats, they condone it indirectly by awarding bonuses and prizes to the stores and departments which turn in the largest profits.

And what does the Kroger Corporation have to lose? After Harter took the Broadway Kroger to court, they were let off with a $20 fine and $15 court costs—less than the cash intake of one minute of business on an average day. Only the consumer loses.

A concerned citizen might wonder about what is happening to the values of this country when a large corporation tacitly encourages cheating the public to squeeze a few more dollars out of their stores. But I worry more about what such a company is doing to its food products to save a few cents here and there and increase the profit margin. Nader's study on the Food and Drug Administration, *The Chemical Feast,* exposed the fact that the FDA does not have the manpower to inspect all phases of food processing and relies upon the large industries to police themselves. Thus, the food companies are fairly free to adulterate their products with more than 9,000 chemicals, 2,000 of which do not even have to be listed on the label. Additives run the gamut of organic and inorganic chemicals including well-known compounds like BHT, BHA, and MSG, and exotics like marine paint remover. Frequently commercial food is ground, dried, boiled, dehydrated, freeze-dried and so over-processed that it loses most of its nutritive value.

It is difficult for the consumer to obtain quality food in the urban areas, and unfortunately it is not very likely that the food companies are going to improve their products in the near future. For many years buying cooperatives have been tried as an alternative to the chain grocery store. Some cities—including Boston, Chicago and Berkeley—have large cooperative stores of many years' stature. However, a new and perhaps more promising form of cooperative is the neighborhood food-buying co-op. The first neighborhood co-ops were organized in Boston and Berkeley in 1967, and were designed so that the residents of a several block area would work together and all reap the benefits. Each week people would put in orders for grains and vegetables, and the volunteers from the neighborhood groups would go to the large wholesale marketplaces and buy the needed items. In Boston, the cooperative was able to start a storefront operation which permitted a member to come in and choose from the meats, grains, and vegetables which were on hand. The Boston cooperative was so successful that it was possible for the organization to start several organic farms.

In Ann Arbor, the cooperatives developed in a pattern somewhat different from the co-ops in Boston and Berkeley. The Rainbow People's Party opened the first cooperative with the purpose of providing fresh vegetables to people at a substantially reduced cost from retail prices. Organizationally, the co-op is very simple. Each week four dollars are collected from the more than 800 members; on Saturday the food is distributed after being purchased that morning at the Detroit Eastern Market. Although this system allows people to receive two bags of groceries very cheaply, the disadvantage is that it does not permit people to choose what they want. An added misfortune is that the Rainbow People's Co-op does not have any legal standing and, therefore, cannot accept food stamps.

In order to expand the available foods beyond the produce handled by the Rainbow People, a broader range cooperative was opened in February 1971. The People's Food Co-op was started by the Open City Co-op in Detroit, which provided the needed capital to rent a counter in the hallway of a boutique and purchase some basic foodstuffs. At first the small co-op dealt only with brown rice and other grains, but in July 1971 it began expanding and moved into a walk-down basement store on State Street. A few weeks later it was incorporated as a nonprofit organization in the State of Michigan with the purpose of "distributing good foods to its members as cheaply as possible, with no individual reaping any financial benefits." At about the same time a fifty-cent membership fee was asked and a plea went out to the community for five-dollar loans to increase the capital reserve of the Co-op. By November the Co-op had more than two thousand members and the capital had been raised to provide yeast, cheese, teas, cider, honey, vegetable oils and an ever-expanding variety of grains and beans.

The People's Co-op on State Street is organized as simply as the Rainbow People's Co-op. Members interested in helping volunteer their time to work in the store, to drive their cars and trucks and pick up food, or to order the needed grains or refined products. Every Tuesday night the membership meets to make policy decisions—how may the Co-op expand, what type of newsletter should be printed, where food should be purchased, and what new items may be available to the Co-op.

Perhaps the most unique feature about the Co-op is that it operates completely on individual honesty. Members come into the store; calculate the cost of the items they wish to purchase according to the wholesale cost which is listed on the bulletin board; and then they add 10 percent to cover Co-op expenses. The 10 percent overhead, which sometimes fluctuates, is applied toward rent, transportation costs, telephone bills and the purchase of brown paper bags. It is also used to accumulate capital for adding new foods, buying an essential mill, and purchasing a much needed truck.

Early in its history the Co-op decided to buy as much organic food as possible and to purchase primarily from the small farmers. With a more than $7,500-per-month capital turnover, the Co-op is a potential boon to the small grower in the Washtenaw County area. The Co-op is growing at a rapid rate—people are discovering that their money goes further at the Co-op, that the food they buy there is unadulterated and nutritious, and that it is enjoyable to be a working part of their own food distribution system. Very shortly the Co-op will outgrow its basement store and be forced to move into a much larger facility. In order for the Co-op to remain a volunteer organization, it will be necessary for it to become a supplier for neighborhood co-ops which will send in orders each week. This plan is now being tested with produce. Each week the members of the neighborhood group submit an itemized list of their vegetable and grain needs to the people whose turn it is to work. Subsequently, they compile the list and on Saturday go down to the central distribution point to pick up the groceries for the whole group. Approximately twice a year each neighborhood group is responsible for working at the central distribution point and providing service to all the neighborhood groups. Through this plan the Co-op will not turn into a large store operation like Kroger, but will maintain a volunteer base and decentralization.

The People's Co-op has become an "organic force" over the past year because of the willingness of people to go to a little extra bother to obtain good quality food. People must put up with some inconveniences such as bringing in their own bottles and jars and hauling produce once or twice a month, but our experience has shown that people enjoy the additional work. Initially only University of Michigan students were interested, but recently large numbers of community people have joined the Co-op. As the Co-op plan unfolds we expect the Kroger and A&P to be covered with cobwebs, and the small organic farmer to be flourishing in the countryside.

THE CAMPUS WHOLE EARTH CO-OP

Jerry Minnich

In Madison, there is room among the 35,000 University of Wisconsin students for the expression of every shade of political philosophy. No movement has come so swiftly, or cut across normal ideological lines so easily, as the environmental movement.

One reason for the movement's fast growth in Madison is the Whole Earth Cooperative—the store where organic gardening meetings are taking place, and a major local center for the environmental struggle.

"This is more than a store," explains Bill Winfield, one of the three innovators of the Co-op. "We have always wanted it to be more than a store, more than just a place to buy things. It is a community center, where anyone can come to try to better his life and his environment."

And Winfield is right. The Co-op does resemble a store in physical appearance, reminiscent of an old-fashioned general store, with its walls paneled in weathered red barn slats, its barewood floors lined with huge barrels of nuts and crocks of whole grains.

But the resemblance to a store is superficial. There are no store owners, no paid clerks, no "customers" in the usual sense, and no profits to be made. A sign on the wall explains, almost apologetically, that a 20 percent mark-up on all foodstuffs is imposed to help cover expenses—but that the markup will go down when sales volume goes up, or when wholesale prices go down. There is no organization to belong to—no co-op membership list, no dues, no red tape.

What there is at the Co-op, in abundance, is involvement. The Whole Earth Learning Community is an integral part of the Co-op, sharing its physical facilities. Here you can sign up for a field trip to discover wild edible plants, or join the natural childbirth discussion group, or attend night classes on the medicinal and healing aspects of herbs and spices.

You can wander in, take a book from the resource library, and read away a rainy afternoon. Chairs and floor pillows are provided for the purpose, and no one will bother you. One group is investigating the possibilities of establishing an industrial cooperative. Others are content in the Sunday birdwatching group. There is no charge for any of the classes or discussion groups.

You can, of course, buy things at the Co-op—mostly books and natural foods. "Our selection is limited right now because we can't really find all the organically-grown foods we want to sell," explains Virginia Lopez, another of the charter organizers. "And we want to be absolutely certain that the organic foods we sell are really organic. We're new in the business, and we want to be sure of our suppliers."

Right now, the Co-op offers a good selection of natural grains and seeds, including oatmeal, rye and whole-wheat flour, corn meal, rolled oats, soybean grits, flaxseed, brown rice, sunflower seeds, lentils and garbanzos. There are barrels of English walnuts and almonds, and in the middle of the store, set on and into an old giant telephone-wire reel, are jars and jars of herbs and spices—Ceylon cinnamon bark, catnip, sassafras bark, kelp, sage, alfalfa, Jamaica ginger, juniper berries, caraway seeds and dried rose hips, among others. On most of the jars there is penciled some pithy advice on how to use the condiments, many of which are new to the young Co-op users. "Good for tea," says one jar. "Put in your bread," advises another.

The selection of foods other than herbs, nuts and grains is limited. Natural honey is sold in large cans, and raw sugar, brewer's yeast, wheat germ, cold-pressed oils, soy sauce, molasses, sea salt and dried fruits are available. A favorite, always quick to sell out, are the roasted, sea-salted soybeans. Fresh produce is sold if a local organic gardener happens to have a surplus and brings it in.

"We really don't want to stock too many foods," says Winfield. "We don't want to become a grocery store, for one thing, and I think it's important to stress the idea that a good life can be lived with a minimum variety of simple, natural foods."

Expansion of the food line will take place this year, however, with the introduction of more fresh organic produce. "We're going to try it," says Ginny Lopez, "but not in a big way. If any of the organic gardeners have surpluses of any crop, they'll donate it and we'll offer it for sale." It will be an informal community effort, as usual.

Plans for the gardening projects are informal, too. Since few of the Co-op users have much gardening space, the Co-op serves as a clearinghouse for free arable land. The city has donated some unused land on the outskirts of town, and a tractor was rented to plow it up last spring. To get a piece of it, all anyone has to do is to dig up three dollars and sign up on the bulletin board. A few local farmers have offered pieces of land for gardening projects, and the university itself provides plots for students who want to grow their own food.

A trip to the university student plots is an experience in itself. On two rolling acres next to the married student apartments, there are hundreds of tiny plots, each no larger than 15 by 10 feet, roped off from their neighbors, and each distinctive. Some have sheets of cheesecloth draped over them, others are covered by makeshift cold frames, and dozens have clanking tin cans and other bird-frightening devices making raucous noises from all directions.

There are the plots of Oriental students, meticulously planned and incredibly manicured—not a weed in sight and not a plant out of place. And there are a few neglected weed patches of those who have lost interest. Some are monocropped—a dozen sweet corn plants or perhaps only tomatoes—while others are veritable sampler plots—one tomato plant, one pepper plant, six carrots, 12 radishes, and one thriving chive purchased at the local supermarket.

Dozens of scarecrows seem to be gathering for a convention on these student plots. Upon entering the area for the first time, your eyes gazing over this mass of paradoxical paraphernalia, you might think that you were in Hong Kong, rather than Madison, Wisconsin. But the old college spirit is there, and the plots are loved. The students race to the gardens after supper every evening to pull the weeds, or lay the mulches, or just to squat and watch miracles springing forth from the earth. This year, more than half the gardens are organic.

Although organic gardening and natural foods are important points of interest at the Co-op, they certainly are not the only ones. Equally important are environmental tools—the knowledge needed to work with the environment, and thus to be able to improve it. This means that any practical knowledge leading to a more natural life, practiced in elemental terms, is a valuable commodity at the Co-op.

These are young people who have grown up with overpowered, gas-spewing automobiles, pop-top bottles, TV dinners, filter-tipped cigarettes, eight-room suburban ranch houses, insecticides, pesticides, and every drug from aspirin to tranquilizers to marijuana. They have been born into wasteful opulence, and they are not impressed with material acquisition. They have rejected materialism as a principle; prefer to return to basics.

Recently at the Co-op, a lecture was given, with illustrative slides, on how to build a log cabin. There are weaving classes, electric welding classes and beadery is taught. There is hope for beginning a pottery shop, and if no class is offered for your particular interest, you can start one by pinning a note on the bulletin board.

Information not available in classes can probably be found in the resource library. Here you'll find books on house-building, basketry, woodworking, knot-tying, cooking, gardening, farming, animal husbandry, beekeeping, camping, and many other practical arts. A favorite is a heavy book called *The Way Things Work*. These young people are determined to learn how to depend on their own resources and knowledge, rather than continuing in a life system in which they are merely pawns in a complex economic system.

Bill Winfield was so impressed by the environmental struggle that he resolved to begin a center for sharing knowledge and environmental tools with others.

With the help of the store's two other organizers, Ginny Lopez and Gerald Young, the Co-op was organized in the late summer of 1969 and opened for business in October.

"We didn't have any money," recalls Bill, "and we had to borrow $1,500 from the Mifflin Street Co-op to get started." The Mifflin Street Co-op is a student-run cooperative grocery store in the traditional Madison student rooming district, on the edge of the campus. Now, after a few years of successful operation, the Mifflin Co-op is the nearest thing to the old general store that Madison has to offer. In both cooperatives, a rare sense of community, which died when Saltines went from barrels into waxwrapped packages, has returned in full flower among Madison's student population.

"We still don't have any money," Bill continues, "but we are serving our purpose. We are open, and we are operating from noon until nine every night except Wednesday."

How does the Co-op pay rent and buy supplies on its low sales volume and slim markup? The answer is on the bulletin board, on the volunteer chart. Co-op users volunteer their help, usually one four-hour block each week, thus virtually eliminating the traditional labor problem for "management." The three organizers of the Co-op receive a token $20 a week for carrying the brunt of the work—keeping books, attending to other management details, and doing more than their share of clerking when volunteers are unavailable. It is obviously a labor of love.

The Co-op's clientele is drawn mainly from the student population. But signs point to a broadening involvement, as more non-students come to see what this center is really like. "The store was located purposely away from the university, in a settled neighborhood," Gerald Young explained to a Milwaukee *Journal* reporter recently. "We want to develop a community feeling here. Many of the customers are students, but older people and couples with young children are beginning to come in."

And, as the Co-op begins to satisfy the curiosity of the resident neighbors, mainly working class people, another group of patrons has begun to make itself known. "We're noticing that some out-of-town people have begun to stop in," says Bill Winfield. "Just the other day a lady from Janesville [41 miles distant] stopped in because Janesville's only health food store closed down." Apparently, the word is spreading among organic gardeners and natural food advocates in neighboring communities, and now they are making it a point to stop by the Co-op on the day they do their weekly shopping in Madison. The coalition of the three—

student environmentalists, resident neighbors, and nearby organic gardeners—just might enable the Whole Earth Co-op to prosper for a long time to come.

HOW TO SET UP AN ORGANIC FOOD CO-OP AT YOUR SCHOOL

Jeff Cox

"How about trying to find out what you would do and be and think and create if there weren't some corporation trying to sell you on doing everything its way," Federal Communications Commissioner Nicholas Johnson suggests.

Applying his suggestion to find good, wholesome food for yourself and your fellow students, you'd probably come up with something close to an organic food conspiracy— which is simply a cooperative buying effort by the students.

Cooperative members by-pass the whole rigamarole of the commercial retail stores: gimmicks, trading stamps, Muzak, hidden costs for advertising, hyped-up and wasteful packaging, chemicalized food that comes from heaven-knows-where and may be heaven-knows-how-old . . . and all the rest of it.

The first thing you need is an organizer, someone who's willing to take charge of the first meeting, at least, and get things rolling.

This nucleus must be well-informed, enthusiastic and . . . here's your first decision . . . either representative of the community as a whole or limited to the student body. The most successful co-ops (at least the ones that have grown the most), usually attempt to include people from all walks of life. The talents of a local lawyer or accountant or truck driver can prove to be worth more than friendship alone.

Call a meeting in someone's home and talk it up. Sooner or later your core group will meet. This is the time to take the steps to incorporate (and where the lawyer comes in handy).

Without incorporation, you'll have the devil's own time trying to rent property, buy equipment and keep your accounts straight. Some states have special laws for incorporating co-ops.

Next you should talk about managers, directors and who's to do the work. If all this sounds like a slavish imitation of the A&P's corporate structure, make up another one. But you'll find that some small but responsible group, with or without rotating membership, is necessary to make the quick, minor decisions that crop up. For instance, your buyers may find a source of beef, but may have to rent a cold locker to store it until distribution day. Somebody has to make a quick decision or you'll lose the source.

You'll also decide at this point how large a cooperative you want. Although the organizing group may be as small as two people, final membership typically runs between 100 and 300 in cities, less than 100 in suburban and country areas. It can be much smaller, and in California you find groups of about 40 people running a food buying service. With such a small group, there's no necessity for renting a storefront and buying cold storage cabinets and all that. Or it can be larger, like the cooperatives discussed earlier. Just about any size will do, but the larger group can afford a more complete line of items. This is because the larger groups have more operating capital with which to snap up a farmer's supply of organic whatever.

Next you'll have to decide how you're going to divvy up the work.

One way of parcelling out the duties is to run a duty roster, just like in the Army. For each job, make a sheet with members' names down one side and days or weeks, as appropriate, across the top. That way you can keep track of who has done what and how often. Per person, it usually doesn't amount to more than an hour or two a week.

The next thing to be considered is the type of financing and charging your group will use. There are options.

In Canada, the most common type of cooperative is the "direct-charge" kind. Under this arrangement, food is sold to the members at cost. The by-laws specify that there is to be no mark-up on food, except a bit for spoilage. Operating expenses, such as rent for a storefront, repairs, supplies, insurance, inventory losses, even salaries if you're into that, are totalled and divided among the members equally, no matter how much food a person buys. This usually comes to no more than $2.50 a week, according to an Ottawa co-op.

That covers the cost of food and operating expenses on

a week-to-week basis, but the co-op also needs a slush fund—enough capital to purchase equipment or special food items. It also allows the co-op to buy with cash and avoid credit, although many co-ops use credit. I think it's something to avoid.

One way in which the Ottawa co-op avoids this is to sell shares to incoming members. Members are required to purchase $10 worth (two shares) when joining and one $5 share quarterly thereafter. If a member leaves the co-op, the corporation buys his shares back from its capital fund.

At the People's Office in Berkeley, California, new members pay a one-time kitty fee of $2—a less complicated arrangement, and one suitable for smaller groups. The larger the group, the more you need a cushion of quite a few thousand dollars. The People's Grocery in Madison started with $1,500 but they all later agreed that $1,500 was cutting it too close.

The advantage of a direct-charge co-op where food is sold at cost and members divvy the operating expenses is that buyers know exactly what they're paying for food. This separates expenses in a handy way for the bookkeepers, also. "At cost" includes any delivery charges and perhaps that little extra for spoilage.

At the Berkeley Food Co-op, the other method—marking up the food—is practiced, with good results. They generally mark up as follows: one cent a pound for items under 10 cents per pound; two cents per pound for items under 20 cents a pound; three cents for items under 30 cents, etc.

A co-op of 300 persons should find operating expenses running somewhat over $600 per week, or slightly more than $2 per member.

There's another type of co-op that's beginning, and which you might consider if your goal is to get wholesome, organic food to students and members of the surrounding communities. The Devcor Farmer-Consumer Co-op, for instance, is part of the International Independence Institute, and plans to help create flourishing markets between organic growers and buyers. As buyers and farmers both contribute toward a capital fund, both are entitled to draw out money to be used for improving farms and homes at one percent interest or less. This makes the food co-op a spark plug for economic gains within cities, and a spur to organic farmers. When the trade is established, Devcor pulls out. If you're interested, write to Devcor, Rt. 1 Box 129, Freeland, Md. 21053.

Only when this preliminary work of organizing is done properly is it time to actually look for food.

You might want to set up a group of two or three members to check out the food co-ops nearest you. Visit them, talk with the principals, find out how they do things and where they're having problems and successes. Nothing will help your effort get off to a smooth start like contact with an already-existed co-op.

During the organizational phase, the buying committee should go to work locating organic farmers as close to campus as possible. One of the reasons co-ops have been so successful in San Francisco is not only the progressive attitude of the city folk, but the tremendous availability of organic food year-round in that locality.

If your school is located in the temperate zones of the upper midwest or east, the winter will pose problems. Large cities, though, such as New York, have farmer's markets. These huge halls of agricultural commerce may have an organic food wholesaler from whom you can buy the usual winter vegetables and food. Check with the largest farm markets in the nearest big city.

Some farmers are strictly organic but don't use the term. When checking with local farmers, you might ask whether they use chemicals and pesticides. Organic is as organic does—despite labels and names.

The Sedgwick Avenue co-op in the Bronx ran into trouble when it started to offer nonfood items to its members. One item offered was toilet paper, but members wanted all different colors and they couldn't get that together. So stick with food, unless you have an unusually amicable group.

Don't forget the large wholesale outlets of organic food such as Walnut Acres. It's not like finding a local farmer, but it's one way to procure rice, other grains and such in bulk, on which you get the bulk break.

Bob Dylan wrote about Daddy in the alley "lookin' for food." You might not have to look as far as the alley, but your buying committee should expect to spend time phoning and driving around. You have to search out sources of supply.

Okay. You've lined up your sources, you know what to buy and how much of it. Your distribution day is Satur-day. What will you need?

You'll need some form of transportation to pick the stuff up and deliver it to the store-front or location you're using as a distribution center. You'll need at least one good scale to measure things out, knives and table space for cutting and wrapping cheese or meat (if you buy parts of carcasses). It's best to have two or three scales if you expect a volume business. Baby scales do fine if you can't find any old Toledoes for sale, reports the Berkeley co-op. You'll also need paper bags and boxes, unless you instruct members to bring their own reusable bags. Labor is much cheaper when volunteered, but the work is difficult enough that you may ultimately want to pay wages.

Timing is essential because food, in hot weather espe-cially, spoils fast. Most co-ops soon rent a store and watch the classifieds for old coolers. A Colorado co-op found two scales, two cold cases and a large freezer for $200, cash and carry.

With proper refrigeration equipment, the distribution is much simpler because you can purchase food as you find it and store it fresh until distribution day. Some developed co-ops, such as the one in Madison, stay open weekdays, and some, like the Berkeley co-op, offer sales to passerby as well as members.

Most likely your co-op won't be selling to the public immediately and you'll find yourself with some damaged and some left over items. One answer is a grand mulligan stew of all the leftovers (but hold the anchovies) served to the people who've manned the co-op on distribution day.

If you've planned wisely and your co-op is an integral part of the campus community, you'll be free of the fabri-cated "necessities" of the mass media and you'll be provid-ing a real service and real food.

There was an editorial in a local newspaper the other day complaining about rising prices. As the editor scoured the countryside of his mind looking for someone to blame it on, his thoughts stuck on consumer groups. "These warlike consumer groups are taking business away from the mass distribution system that American business has developed. This drives up prices. We need to return to the efficiency of the large chain stores. We don't need less goods, we need more super markets," our newspaper editor opined.

Doesn't talk like that make you want to start your own food conspiracy?

BRIEFLY . . .

The essential steps for beginning a cooperative include:

1) Begin small with several basic foodstuffs that people need, and then gradually expand as more capital becomes available.
2) Make people aware of the different qualities of foods and the different sources of foods.
3) Recruit volunteers to work from people who have time and are concerned about the quality of food they are buying in the supermarket.
4) Learn about buying organic foods and find organic farmers who will sell directly to the Co-op in the area.
5) Work to reduce transportation costs by finding local sources for different kinds of foods.
6) Incorporate as a nonprofit organization.

FOOD CO-OPS AND BUYING CLUBS

Alternative Distributing
2366 Telegraph
North of Bay Area
Berkeley, CA 94702

Organic Food Conspiracy
Alison Farley
2326 Sacramento
Berkeley, CA 94702

People's Union Co-op Farm
J. C. Crampton
8734 W. Manning
Fresno, CA

Free Venice Food Co-op
Don Lubin
31 Breeze Ave.
Los Angeles, CA 90291

Pacific Husbandry
John Bennett
845 via de la Paz No. 14
Pacific Palisades, CA 90272

Consumer Co-op
Robert Broh
164 S. California Ave.
Palo Alto, CA 94306

Lorraine Klevansky
1285 Dale Ave., Mt. View
Palo Alto, CA 94306

Consumers Co-op of Berkeley
Don Rothenberg
4805 Central Ave.
Richmond, CA 94804

Wayne McCracken
1649 7th Ave.
San Diego, CA

Haight-Ashbury Co-op
Loretta O'Sullivan
165 Belvedere
San Francisco, CA 94117

Noe Valley
Ralph Gallagher
418 Valley
San Francisco, CA 94131

Consumers Co-op
Bob Intersimone
2115 N. Pacific Ave.
Santa Cruz, CA 95060

Natural Foods Store Co-op
Wendy Kaysing
P.O. Box 371
West Point, CA 95255

Boulder Food Co-op
Mark Gunther
1227 Walnut
Boulder, CO 80302

The Food Co-op
1100 Champa St.
Denver, CO 80204

New Haven Food Co-op
457 Greenwich Ave. No. 1
New Haven, CT 06519

Alternative Vittles
Stan Altland
1478 Gulf to Bay
Clearwater, FL 33515

Sunflower
The Sarasota Food Store
1549 Main St.
Sarasota, FL 33577

Fed. of Southern Co-ops
Don Speicher
52 Fairlie St., N.W.
Atlanta, GA 30303

New Morning Food Co-op
862 Rosedale
Atlanta, GA 30306

Kokua Country Food Store
2357 S. Beretaina St.
Honolulu, HI 96814

People Not Profits
Steve Morris
Nuama House
2930 Nuama Rd.
Honolulu, HI 96819

Way Inn Co-op
P.O. Box 527
Kealakekua, HI 96750

Hyde Park Co-op
Gladys Scott
55th & Lake Park
Chicago, IL 60637

La Gente Food Co-op
3227 N. Halstead
Chicago, IL 60657

D. H. Wheat Food Co-op
Third Unitarian Church
301 N. Mayfield Ave.
Chicago, IL 60644

People's Pantry
Bob Bucher
402 W. Main
N. Manchester, IN 46962

New Pioneer Co-op Society
518 Bowery St.
Iowa City, IO 52240

Food Buying Co-op
c/o Dave Davis
Univ. & Community Resource
   Council
100 E. Annex, Univ. of Maine
Orono, ME 04473

Glut Washington Food
405 34th St.
Mt. Rainer, MD 20822

Yellow Sun Natural Foods Co-op
Augie Cohn
35 N. Pleasant St.
Amherst, MA 01002

Arlington Food Co-op
Peter Callaterra
38 Bartlett Ave.
Arlington, MA 02174

Athol Peoples Food Co-op
Ed Bruno
216 Exchange St.
Athol, MA 01331

Beverly Co-op
Nick McAuliffe
NSCAC 356R Cabot St.
Beverly, MA 01915

Interfaith Food & Grain
George Whitehouse
490 Beacon St.
Boston, MA 02115

Peace and Beans
Jill Dardick
522 Commonwealth Ave.
Boston, MA 02215

South End Food Co-op
Karen Crestman/Mary Ann
c/o Help Program
Boston, MA 02216

Student Union Food Co-op
Matthew Reich
12 Babbitt St.
Boston, MA 02215

Beansprout II
Charles Lerrige
80 Nottonghill Rd.
Brighton, MA 02135

Beansprout I
Joyce Thompson
12 Douglas St.
Cambridge, MA 02139

Cambridge Central Food Co-op
Ken Alper
3 Clinton St. No. 4
Cambridge, MA 02139

Cambridge Food Co-ops
Red Book
91 River St.
Cambridge, MA 02139

Cambridgeport Food Co-op
Holly Sue Angier
65 Pleasant St.
Cambridge, MA 02139

Franklin St. Food Co-op
438 Franklin St.
Cambridge, MA 02139

Hancock Street Food Co-op
Henry Smilowitz
Cambridge, MA 02139

Pearl Street Co-op
Regina Flaherty
53 Pearl St.
Cambridge, MA 02139

Good Food Union
Woolman Hill
Deerfield, MA 01342

Yarmouth Co-op
Box 379
Dennisport, MA 02639

The People First Food Co-op
Kevin Cumming
238 Bowdoin St.
Dorchester, MA 02122

Brandywine Village Co-op
Debby Leiberman
42 Trustman Terr.
East Boston, MA 02128

Another Day Co-op
52 Maple St.
Florence, MA 01060

Haverhill Food Co-op
Allen Carbello
Able Comm. Action Center
5 Vine St.
Haverhill, MA 01830

Free Co-op
Leonie Flannery
22 Vine St.
Lexington, MA 02173

Lexington Food Co-op
Leah Vetter
30 Woodcliff Rd.
Lexington, MA 02173

Lowell Food Co-op
Miles Rappoport
6 Boynton Terr.
Lynn, MA 01902

Scituate Food Co-op
Phillis Mettauer
435 Tilden Rd.
N. Scituate, MA 02060

Mission Hill
John Osberg
53 Wesley St.
Roxbury, MA 02120

Columbia Pt. Food Assoc.
20 Montpelier Rd.
Columbia Pt.
South Boston, MA 02111

Weston Organic Co-op
Sheila Denny-Brown
87 Spruce Hill Rd.
Weston, MA 02193

Hard Times Food Co-op
Anthony Teso
270 Pleasant St.
Worcester, MA 01609

Worcester Food Co-op
Louise Hagen
9 Larch St.
Worcester, MA 01609

Grain Train Co-op
Rt. 1, Box 60
Petoskey, MI 49770

Prairie Dog Store
Univ. of Minn.
Marshall, MN 56258

Ecology Co-op
1023 Eighth St. S.E.
Minneapolis, MN 55414

Mill City Food
c/o N. Country Co-op
26th & Bloomington
Minneapolis, MN 55404

North Country Food Co-op
Keith and Dean
2129 Riverside
Minneapolis, MN 55404

Whole Foods
2502 1st Ave.
Minneapolis, MN 55404

St. Paul Co-op
996 Selby Ave.
St. Paul, MN 55102

Columbia Foods Co-op
Mark Valburn
915 E. Broadway
Columbia, MO 65201

Community Food Conspiracy
3800 McGee St.
Kansas City, MO 64109

New England Peoples Co-op
South Co-op
52 Main St.
W. Lebanon, NH 03784

N.J. Natural Food & Farm Co-op
216 Belmont Ave.
Ocean, NJ 12202

Manager
Off Center
72 State St.
Binghamton, NY 13905

Brockport Co-op
Debbie Kirsten
181 Utica St.
Brockport, NY 14420

Allentown Food Co-op
226 Maryland
Buffalo, NY 14201

Lexington Food Co-op
Lori Rivard/Leslie
    Benthermueller
Paul Spencer
224 Lexington Ave.
Buffalo, NY 14222

N. Buffalo Co-op
3225 Main
Buffalo, NY 14214

Grocery Co-op
Lois Proiette
7 Whitaker Rd.
Fulton, NY 13069

Organic Energy
68-06 Fresh Meadow Lane
Fresh Meadows, NY 11365

Geneva Food Co-op
Bvent Bleier
561 S. Main St.
Geneva, NY 14456

People's Town Hall Food Co-op
John Brush
488 New York Ave.
Huntington, NY 11743

Natural Foods Co-op
Josh Valente
12 S. Second Ave.
Mt. Vernon, NY 10550

Real Food Co-op
c/o Open House
412 Linn St.
Ithaca, NY 14850

Real Food Store
53 Main St.
New Paltz, NY 12561

Broadway Local Food Co-op
John Mack/Mary Roby
615 W. 164th St. Apt. 51-D
New York, NY 10025

Greenhouse Association
466 Amsterdam Ave.
New York, NY 10024

Wild Rice Co.
154 W. 17th St.
New York, NY 10011

Syracuse Community Food Co-op
Linda Reed
278 Genesee Pk. Dr.
Syracuse, NY 13200

Troy Peoples Co-op
Claire Frankel
279 Hoosick St.
Troy, NY 12180

Trumansburg Food Co-op
Carl Mansdorf/Mary Litke
46 South St.
Trumansburg, NY 14886

Chapel Hill Food Co-op
Charles Jeffries
501 E. Rosemary St.
Chapel Hill, NC 27514

Peoples Intergalactic Food
Conspiracy No. 1
Jon Carmel
5091 D. S.
Durham, NC 27703

Tocchi Foods
303 Roberts St.
Fargo, ND 58102

Harvey Forstag
OSU Food Co-op
2377 N. Fourth St.
Columbus, OH 43201

Raccoon Valley Food Friends
Ann Hagedorn
17 Samson Pl.
Granville, OH 43023

Jeanne Owings
Kent Food Co-op
228 Gougler Ave.
Kent, OH 44240

Real Good Food Co-op
Antioch College Union
Yellow Springs, OH 43710

Ashland Food Co-op
88 N. Main
Ashland, OR 97520

Forest Acres Co-op
3362 Table Rock Rd.
Central Point, OR 97501

Grower's Market
301 Lincoln
Eugene, OR 97401

Willamette People's Co-op
1391 22nd E.
Eugene, OR 97403

Salem Comm. Food Store
1190 12th St. S. E.
Salem, OR 97302

Emily Food Co-op
4930 Coyote Creek
Wolf Creek, OR 97497

Nashua Food Co-op
Gail Morrison
7 Gordon St.
Hudson, NH 03051

Anthony Auretto
Dept. of I.E.
Lehigh Univ.
Bethlehem, PA 18015

Comm. Food Co-op of W. Phila.
c/o Andy Stern
3907 Spruce St.
Philadelphia, PA 19104

Harriet Fleischman
c/o W. Oak Lane Co-op
6738 Old York Rd.
Philadelphia, PA 19126

Carol Henningsen
c/o Germantown People's Food
3207 W. Penn. St.
Philadelphia, PA 19144

Dick Hiler
Parkway Program
Community Gamma
16 N. Front
Philadelphia, PA 19106

Jim Markunas
c/o Concerned Neighborhood
   Co-op
St. Davids Episcopal Church
481 Flamingo St.
Philadelphia, PA 19128

Brown Student Food Co-op
90 Waterman St.
Providence, RI 02906

Harvest Moon Foods
100 W. Main St.
Vermillion, SD 57069

Texas Food Co-ops
Roger Pierce
222 Varsity Circle
Arlington, TX 76013

Austin Consumer's Co-op
319 Texas Union
Austin, TX 78712

Debbie Monas
Austin Food Co-op
2115 W. 10th St.
Austin, TX 78703

People Buying Together
3335 Inwood
Dallas, TX 75235

Steve Frank
192 N. Willard St.
Burlington, VT 05401

New England Peoples Co-op
North Co-op
160 N. Winooski Ave.
Burlington, VT 05401

Westburke Collective
Box 62
Westburke, VT 05871

Robert Dressel
Eastern Co-ops, Inc.
7758 Donnybrook Ct.
Annandale, VA 22003

The Store
1919 W. 2nd
Spokane, WA 99204

West Side Co-op
602 Water St.
Eau Claire, WI 54701

Common Market
Elaine Nesterick
1340 E. Washington Ave.
Madison, WI 53703

Mifflin St. Grocery Co-op
32 N. Bassett St.
Madison, WI 53703

Whole Earth Grainery & Truck
   Store
111 Ivinson Ave.
Laramie, WY 82070

CHAPTER V

ORGANIC FOODS IN THE CAFETERIA

"There's a quiet revolution going on at colleges around the nation. It's a revolution against mushy vegetables, mystery meat and the foods students have accepted for so many years. The revolution is in university food services."

M. C. Goldman and Rich Meislin

College campus cafeterias that up to now have offered only conventional "plastic" meals are likely to find themselves in the middle of a new clamor for natural eating and better foods. Students at several West Coast schools launched the organic-food-in-the-cafeteria movement, and the trend is advancing eastward in giant strides.

A large share of the inspiration comes from developments such as the one at the University of California at Santa Cruz, where a student garden project swelled into insistence that the organic foods they were growing be made available in an "alternative choice" cafeteria line. Now several years old, the project is still expanding and has consistently drawn upwards of 40 percent of the campus eaters into the organic food line—with many others crossing over to get the better bread.

More recently, the University of California, Davis campus cafeteria started offering natural foods. Carolyn Krauss was the moving force behind the Davis kitchen, organizing a drive for student signatures to present to the university's catering service. It took about three months and then a lot of work to open a closed-off wing of the cafeteria, where volunteers now prepare and serve organic dinners to about 100 students a day.

Taking his cue from the Davis success, Bob Warren sparked a campaign at Sacramento State College. Warren believes in organic foods as a way of life. He says he isn't trying to convert people to his way of eating, but feels that those who like natural foods should get what they want on the college campus. So he began a drive to get organic foods served in the cafeteria by setting up petition stands to enlist the 1,000 signatures needed to bring it to the student senate.

In the East, a classroom nutrition seminar at New College in Sarasota, Florida, led students to seek a change in the college dining room bill-of-fare. They've succeeded—and some of them are growing vegetables organically to help supply the better menu. A similar evolution is taking place at Florida Presbyterian College in St. Petersburg. The manager of the food service volunteered to provide one student the fruit and nuts he wished to include as a major part of his diet. Then another student, who had worked at a health resort, asked if he could switch to the same program. From there on, student interest mushroomed. More and more of the student body showed a preference for the natural foods program which was expanded to include cereals, juices, eggs and nut butter. Now 360 students (out of a college enrollment of 900) are in the natural foods program. Some interesting effects on those participating: better weight control, fewer colds, improved complexions, and—because they feel so good—much less use of drugs or stimulants.

Some of this nation's most prestigious colleges are offering students a natural food alternative and the students are literally eating it up.

Yale University in New Haven, Connecticut, is a good example. The school began a natural foods line in its Commons Dining Hall late in 1971, and everyone—students and kitchen staff alike—seems to be benefiting from the move.

"The impetus for us to start our natural foods line at Yale came primarily from our students," Albert E. Dobie, manager of Yale food services said. "As we sat down and talked to students about special problems and special diets, it began to seem that it would be a good idea."

Helen Doherty, dietician for the Massachusetts Institute of Technology in Cambridge, Massachusetts, had a similar story to tell. "We're not completely organic," she said, "so we're calling our line a natural foods line. But we do try to have organic grains, seeds and beans as much as possible."

MIT had an even better reason than Yale to go along with the tide of food consciousness among students today—

young people attending the university have no obligation to eat in the dining halls, and to get them to eat there, the food service had to find a new and better selling point. Natural foods appear to have been a good answer.

Miss Doherty admits she had problems getting used to the new foods—"I'm so commercially oriented," she said— but now she enjoys it. Beatrice Trum Hunter's *Natural Foods Cookbook* has become the Bible of the cooks, and they always have an eye out for new and interesting recipes for their patrons.

"I'd never sprouted a bean in my whole life," Miss Doherty explained with a chuckle. "Now we have them sprouting in every available space." The first few days of the new service—in the beginning of February—were disappointing. "The brown rice the first two nights was horrible —mushy and sticky," Miss Doherty said. "Now we've got that down. We cook our vegetables without butter and salt, and a few people complain that they're too bland. But we just tell them to put their own salt and butter on if they want it—and most people like it the way it is."

Like Yale's, MIT's new program has received a good amount of feedback from student diners—in fact, said Miss Doherty, "the best feedback of any project we've undertaken." And, in the spirit of the natural foods movement, there's good interaction between dining service and student. For example, Miss Doherty said, "the first time we were going to serve dry unsulfured fruits, we felt that they were so unsightly that we had to serve them stewed or in some kind of dish where they could be disguised. So we did that, and students said they would rather have them raw. We're experimenting with dishes and inventing some as we go along."

Also in line with the movement to make consumers aware of what is in the foods they eat, MIT food services issues a detailed listing of the ingredients in each new dish that it serves. This way, vegetarians can more easily pick out the things they might not want to eat and everyone knows exactly what they're getting in their meals.

MIT also had a considerable amount of trouble finding suppliers for many of its basic foods. But people involved in the natural foods movement are always willing to help others who are interested, and Miss Doherty was surprised and pleased by the responses she received from local merchants. "Everyone you meet is willing to help you, and everyone who's already into the natural foods idea is willing to help you get into it too," she said.

Many of MIT's supplies now come from New England merchants, with Corners of the Mouth in Cambridge—a local organic foods restaurant and bakery—supplying organic whole wheat breads, and Erewhon Trading Company —one of the nation's largest organic suppliers—shipping grains to MIT from its Boston offices.

For those students not fortunate enough to have organic or natural foods served in their school dining halls, alternatives exist. Organic food restaurants are booming near several campuses, and organic food co-ops among students are not unknown.

But one of the most novel ways of peddling organic wares has been started in Boston by Matthew Chait, an enthusiastic organic vegetarian. On sunny days, Matthew Chait's Ricycles—organic food vending carts attached to bicycles—can be spotted near many of the area's colleges and universities. In fact, the sight of students crowding the Ricycles instead of the university dining halls is a factor which led to MIT's entry into the natural foods field.

Ricycle fare generally includes a cooked grain or rice dish, a vegetable course, soup, whole grain organic bread, hot organic cider or tea and dessert—and only $1 buys a combination plate.

But the food scene at colleges is not all glowing. Mushy vegetables, processed and canned foods, thick fatty gravies and other non-nutritional gunk still remains the only meal choice at many schools. And some are practicing a natural foods tokenism which falls just short of outright deception.

Harvard University, for example, one of the nation's most respected academic institutions, instituted in 1972 "basic foods" tables in all of its dining halls. Rolled oats, wheat germ, raisins, eggs, honey, yogurt, peanut butter and cottage cheese peer from gleaming stainless steel bowls at each meal. But things are not always as they seem. Investigation revealed that the peanut butter was hydrogenated, the raisins were sulfured, the cottage cheese was processed, and the oats were not organic and the eggs were neither organic nor fertile. (The yogurt, however, was fine, provided by one of the few manufacturers who do not use additives.)

Harvard's lead reportedly will be followed in the near future by Tufts, and undoubtedly will be far more widespread than the better routes of MIT and Yale. Most Harvard students who patronize the basic foods tables, which were originally described by The Harvard *Crimson,* the university newspaper, as a concession to "health food nuts," do not appear to know about the actual quality of the foods found there. Nor do they seem to care. "The food here is so starchy that you begin to realize you're going to be hungry a few hours later. So I go to the basic foods table and fill up on that. At least it's got *some* substance to it," one student explained.

Another Harvard student, an organic vegetarian, moved out of the university housing system to a cooperative house in order to break his food contract. He had taken his complaint through the entire ladder of appropriate officials, having his hopes alternately raised and shattered, and finally was told that he would be unable to "get off board" without leaving his dorm. The explanation given was that his breaking his food contract would set a poor precedent, enabling more students to leave the university dining halls and undermining the economic foundation of the food services.

"The counterculture is affecting the attitudes and values of many teen-agers in regard to food," said Ruth L. Huenemann, a University of California nutrition expert.

Although it's unlikely that a counterculture cuisine of carrot juice and wheat germ will replace cola drinks and chocolate bars in the stomachs of most teen-agers, Dr. Huenemann said, "there's a shift away from highly-refined foods like candy and soft drinks. Your counterculture kids are eating fewer empty calories."

Dr. Huenemann, at a nutrition-education conference in Washington, said she thought the movement toward organic foods "could have a good effect on our culture," but she took issue with some dietary habits. "Some of the things they're doing are not nutritional," she said. "Where they try to live on cereal alone, as a nutritionist, I cannot condone this. However, with a combination of cereal and legumes—dried peas, dried beans and lentils—you are able to get all the amino acids you need."

Discussing the value of food grown organically, Dr. Huenemann said: "Some of your organically-grown fruits and vegetables have slight nutritional benefits. The distance from the field to the table may be shorter. You may have less vitamin loss from storage. Also, they may have been grown more slowly because they're not heavily irrigated or fed with as much fertilizer," techniques often used to make food grow faster. "Therefore, they may have less water content and more flavor."

Dr. Huenemann said she thinks the organic food movement will continue to spread. "A shift away from our over-consumption has to come," she said. There has to be some modification of our wasteful way of life. The counterculture movement's interest in organic food may make a contribution to that effect.

Will more colleges and universities start hearing from students who want natural food? There's no doubt about it. The call reflects a genuine, wholesome aspect of the total environmental awareness today's young people continue to demonstrate—starting with themselves. The prospect is encouraging as well as significant. Would that their enthusiasm and the momentum of what's happening on campus help penetrate the complacency stubbornly remaining in so many other people and places!

CHAPTER VI

ORGANIC AGRICULTURE AND THE LAND GRANT COLLEGES

Robert Rodale

In my opinion, the land grant colleges have helped to foul up this country by applying too many simplistic technological remedies to farm problems without trying to foresee the eventual consequences of those remedies. Workers at the land grant colleges have continually used advancing technology to replace human hands with machines, chemicals, and special varieties of crop plants. The result has been more food produced by each farmer and on each acre, but at the same time much displacement of people to the cities, high costs for welfare, other social disruption, and often sad environmental consequences.

In using the power of advancing technology in such blind ways, the land grant colleges and their allies—the chemical and machinery firms—have not done things differently than other segments of industry. Almost all phases of American life for the past 100 years have been characterized by such technological penetration, with little thought for what is likely to happen beyond this year's profit and loss statement. The automobile industry is a perfect example. All it appears to be concerned about is the production of more cars each year, plus the making of more highways on which those cars can travel. The basic question of how people can transport themselves in the most environmentally sound, economical and satisfying ways appears not to be the concern of the auto industry. That is a problem for someone else to solve, they seem to say.

Food is another example. Technology, blindly applied, has given Americans a fantastic range of convenience food—and nutritional problems that were not dreamed of before the advent of that technology. The same kind of indictment can be—and has been—made of many other facets of American life, and steps are now being taken to try to correct those problems.

I believe, however, that the problem of wrong use of technological remedies is more serious in agriculture than in industry and other phases of life, and merits special attention. There are several reasons:

1. The government, through the land grant colleges, has been the primary agent for this technological disruption of our lives and environment. Therefore, government has a special reason to try to set things right. Also, because the land grant colleges are under government control to a large extent, the means for changing the direction of their work exists.

2. Agriculture, rooted in our fertile soils, is the basic source of American strength. Technological mistakes and the disruption of our farm population sets the stage for a serious long-term threat to our nation's health. The technological manipulation of our agriculture is a perfect example of the all-too-human trait of putting short-term profits before the obligation to maintain resources for long-term use. Chemical agribusiness is not proven as a long-term technique. It is still experimental.

3. Finally, the vast rural lands of America have traditionally been a refuge for our troubled citizens, seeking new opportunities and a new start in life. The present system of farming, oriented to big business, has effectively closed off that alternative for millions of people, and will shut it off entirely for all but a handful of farmers if the present trends continue. If that happens, one of our most precious social resources will have been lost, replaced by urban ghettos of the most miserable kind.

Organic gardeners and farmers are the remnants of the many millions of people who at one time constituted the yeoman core of American stability and strength. We are largely the little people still living on the land, not the businessmen farmers. We grow vegetables and fruits on small plots, using natural and non-chemical methods because we have found by experience that those methods are very effective. We concentrate on building the fertility of the soil, because we know that a fertile soil produces abundant crops with much less work and expense than a depleted soil.

There are some farmers in our organic group, and more are joining every day, but in the farm country we are still a tiny minority.

The amount of help that the land grant colleges have given to the organically oriented people over the years is hardly large enough to be worth mentioning. Some of the techniques of modern, conventional gardening and agriculture are used on organic gardens and farms. Improved tractors and tillers are a help, and so are the new biological controls for insects. But the great bulk of new chemicals and machines and ideas coming out of the land grant colleges have been anti-organic in their orientation, and of no use to us.

The real tragedy is that the agriculture colleges have often attacked the organic people—who really are the only farmers and gardeners completely in tune with the environment—simply to create a smoke-screen to mask the stupidity of their own technological policies. We are the kooks and the nuts, they say, while their chemical-spraying farmer, sitting on his mammoth tractor, is supposedly nature's nobleman, wisely following their scientific instructions to the letter.

Without really knowing what organic growing techniques are, and with even less knowledge of how to use them, they repeat the bald statement that millions of people would starve if organic farming were universal.

The real truth, which these land grant college scientists don't want to face, is that if organic systems were used universally in agriculture and in urban life, our country would be much better fed and stronger in many ways. But you cannot just take the chemicals away from conventional farmers and expect them to become effective organic farmers overnight. You must have a plan, and do many things in an organized way.

Garbage, sewage and other organic wastes must be returned to the land instead of being burned or buried. That would solve an important urban problem.

Displaced farm workers now living in cities must be given the chance to return to the land with dignity, working their own small plots of land where they can support themselves. That would save billions of dollars in welfare costs.

Most importantly, the land grant colleges must use their

scientific resources to create a new generation of what I call the soft technology of farming. They must create machines and techniques that are better and smaller at the same time, instead of concentrating on large-scale techniques that always end up replacing people. We organic people do not want to go back to the old ways. We are not advocating a return to primitive farming, where people are worn out by hard work by the time they are 40. We want a new, ecologically-oriented agriculture that can be made possible by the intelligent application of the best scientific thinking to our problems.

Here are some of the areas in which scientific effort is needed:

1. Energy. Conventional farm technology is essentially slanted toward making the farmer an agent in the use of stored solar energy (in the form of processed coal, oil, gas and soluble fertilizer deposits) for the increased production of crops and animals. By contrast, all farming prior to 100 years ago, and organic farming today, operates primarily on current solar energy falling on crop lands.

Absorption and conversion of current solar energy is far from complete using present methods. Through photosynthesis, plants convert only a small fraction of sun energy into usable food. By extending the growing season through natural means, ways can be found to increase the conversion rate of current solar energy on small farms. More intensive methods for growing fruits and vegetables also make much more efficient use of the sun's energy than does the growing of most farm crops, such as wheat, corn and soybeans.

With new technology based on more scientific input, sun energy can also be used on small farms for home heating, waste conversion, and increased movement of water from the subsoil to the surface, by way of deep-rooting plants. Also very interesting is the culture of semi-tropical fish (eating low-priced grass as food) in solar-heated dome structures.

Other sources of energy can be tapped for small-farm use. Wind-power generation can be perfected, and organic wastes can be used to produce methane gas for heating, lighting, and even for powering of automobiles. Power storage systems suited for small-farm use can also be developed.

2. Waste conversion and fertilizer production. Ways can be developed to make many waste products of urban living into valuable fertilizers, with less labor and handling than is currently needed. Present technology is adequate to convert almost any organic waste to a fertilizer or soil-conditioner, but process-costs need to be reduced. Also, subsidies by urban government seeking to dispose of wastes should be directed to small, organic farms.

3. Machinery. Agricultural engineering departments of land grant colleges should cease work (at taxpayers' expense) on machines for large farms and work only on machines that will make small farming more practical and competitive. The rotary tiller is such a machine. Using small power units, it enables large-scale gardeners to do a thorough job of tilling the soil. It is essentially a miniaturization of the traditional plowharrow machines.

Similar miniaturizations of all farm machines are needed. Some are already available, particularly tractors and related equipment. But work is needed to develop miniaturized harvesting equipment oriented toward making individual farm workers able to compete with large-scale machines.

4. Biological insect control. Much good work has already been done toward finding natural substitutes for toxic chemicals pesticides, thanks to both the ecology movement and the realization some years back that pesticides are too expensive and have a limited useful life because of the build-up of insect resistance.

Increased scientific efforts in the biological control area are necessary. Of great interest are recent discoveries indicating that plants, animals and insects (and perhaps even man) are tied together in a chemical communication network. The active agents of this network are pheromones, essentially airborne or waterborne hormones. Pheromones provide the answer to many questions that have puzzled both biologists and farmers, and point toward new culture methods that eliminate toxic risks and lower costs of production. However, chemical pesticides cover up or interfere with the pheromone network, so the system of natural food production is not always compatible with partial use of chemicals, as in integrated control.

5. Educational technology. Thorough studies should

be made of all ways in which both city and farm people could be taught to appreciate the virtues of small-scale production. Present education practices are directed toward creating agricultural specialists, or people motivated toward working in agribusiness operations.

6. Marketing techniques. Here is an area of great potential benefit for the small-farm movement. Intensive scientific and business efforts should be directed toward perfecting methods of getting fresh, relatively unprocessed food quickly and cheaply from farm to consumer. Cooperatives can be of help. So can improved packaging and shipping techniques.

On a recent visit to the U.S. Department of Agriculture, an editorial associate of mine requested that the USDA set up an "organic farming office" that would distribute useful information about managing a small farm by organic methods—for example, the cheapest ways to spread manure over fields; mechanical ways to control weeds; biological insect controls for the small farm; resistant varieties, and other subjects which the USDA obviously knows much about, but which farmers are not being informed about regularly by extension agents. Even a one-man office would be a start toward recognition by the USDA and land grant colleges that organic farmers are, in fact, a legitimate constituency to serve.

The request was turned down however, since—in the opinion of the USDA official—the Department already served not only all *farmers* but all *Americans*. The USDA and the land grant college complex have something for everyone, his reply went on, including organic farmers.

But over the years, everyone has come to be spelled with a capital E, and USDA policies reflect the recognition that agriculture is a Business also spelled with a big B. Evidently in the millions of dollars spent annually, there isn't much money or time left over to aid the family farmer —and certainly not the organic family farmer.

A continuation of present land grant college actions and philosophy will insure that there is no alternative to the destructive course of U.S. agriculture. Farms will get fewer and fewer, and farming profits will go to bigger and bigger conglomerates. More and more people—who want to remain on the land—will find their own tax dollars used to fight against the very agricultural alternative they are trying to create.

Right now, a sizable number of American consumers are paying a subsidy for foods grown by organic farmers. When you think about it, these Americans are being taxed twice in effect. First, all their regular tax dollars go through government channels to support and perpetuate chemicalized, agribusiness food production. Second, they are paying—voluntarily, I admit—an additional subsidy to encourage farmers to change away from methods which their official tax dollars support.

Existing efforts of land grant colleges are clearly not enough. Constructive programs will only develop when land grant college advisory committees and policies aggressively seek to develop the ways and means to help solve the problems plaguing family farmers and the people in rural communities. Half-hearted efforts—as we have seen in the past —get us nowhere. We need people in official capacities in the USDA and land grant colleges to say: "I am ready and able to support specific research and programs which will help more people make a better living on the farm. . . . I am ready and able to support specific alternatives to our present agricultural system."

This does not mean a condemnation of everything now going on in the agricultural system. This does not mean to be a call to stop all projects and issue statements like "We can do it, but you must pick which half of the U.S. will starve to death."

All I am saying is that those who seek change should have official recognition . . . should have a substantial amount of the dollars now being expended to support constructive change . . . and that people in high places should not be so quick to condemn those who would alter the agricultural status quo.

Through my involvement with ORGANIC GARDENING AND FARMING magazine, I am most familiar with the agricultural alternatives offered by the organic method. This is only one of the terms and forces now developing. I am sure that other labels and other terms will develop.

But we are witnessing a very vital development taking place around the identifying label offered by the word "organic." It has come to stand for an attitude that looks upon smallness as a virtue. In an era when most city people have grown up without any personal communication with the producer of their foods, the organic route is clearly different. Suddenly, the consumer can identify the farmer, and the farmer can identify the personal needs of the consumer. No longer is the supermarket clerk or the television commercial the most vivid contact. Suddenly, the organic family farmer replaces the jolly Green Giant.

The word "organic" is helping city people to understand farming problems. The word is helping to forge an alliance between farmers and consumers. A great part of our present problems in society is due to programs that have actually built walls around farms and cities—programs that have isolated one segment of our society from another. This separation means that representatives of city voters vote against farm-oriented programs, and vice versa. Wouldn't it be great if more programs and alternatives stressed the common benefits to both city and rural people?

I ask the land grant college system to look upon the needs of organic farmers and organic food customers as a step toward developing future programs which that system could develop. These people want to tear down the barriers to communication. These people are against the present trend where farmers go indifferently in one direction, while consumers go in the other—each blaming the other for their respective troubles.

There should develop a clear recognition that the purpose of the land grant college system is not to create only one single agricultural system that helps only those who are big enough to plug into it. Diversity is a healthy characteristic of all environments. And we need a land grant college system that thrives on diversity.

Recently, our company sponsored a National Conference on Organic Farming and Composting to report on how cities are using—and can use—organic wastes like sewage sludge to build soils, and how the world needed an agricultural system that makes use of those organic wastes. We believe organic farming can provide such an agricultural system. Organic farming can provide high-quality food to consumers in nearby cities, farms that can provide jobs, farms that can be both economically- and environmentally-sound. And farms that can use composted city wastes to build humus into soils.

The Conference brought together qualified experts in

solid waste management and public health, but we were unable to secure a single representative from the land grant colleges to present a report on those topics. As has been the case with the development of organic agriculture in this country, it continues to be the responsibility of proponents of an organic agriculture to be their own researchers, their own experimenters, their own extension services—while the tax-supported research into agribusiness goes on and on.

Our Conference was most fortunate to have Wendell Berry—this year's Distinguished Professor at the University of Kentucky and an organic farmer—as the transition speaker to shift the meeting from an urban orientation with wastes to an agricultural emphasis on organic food growing. His topic was "Where Cities and Farms Come Together," and he began this way:

"The mentality of organic agriculture is not a technological mentality—though it concerns itself with technology. It does not merely ask what is the easiest and cheapest and quickest way to reach an immediate aim. It is, rather, a complex and radical attitude toward the problem of our relation to the earth. It is concerned with the long-term question of what humans need from the earth, and what duties and devotions humans owe the earth in return for the satisfaction of their needs. It understands that the terms of a lasting agriculture are not human terms, that the final terms are nature's, that an agriculture—and for that matter, a culture—that holds in ignorance or contempt the truths and the mysteries of nature is doomed to failure, for it is out of control.

"At least since the time of Henry Adams, numerous critics and historians have been concerned with the disintegration of the synthesis of disciplines that made the medieval cathedral one of the supreme articulations of humanity's relation to God. Only recently have we begun to be aware of the disintegration of an even more ancient and fundamental synthesis—that of the old peasant and yeoman agriculture, which still stands as the best articulation of humanity's relation to the world. This was not simply an agriculture; at best, it was also a *culture* of such deep-rooted and complex wisdom that it preserved the fertility of the earth under the most intensive human use. It was a culture that made men the preservers rather than the parasites of the sources of their life. The organic movement has its roots in this ancient agriculture that was so wise and profound a bond between human beings and their fields. And it is the rise of the organic movement that affords us a perspective from which we can understand the consequences of the disintegration of that bond—a disintegration that now palpably threatens the destruction, not merely of human culture, but of human life as well."

Professor Berry then went on to describe the forces that have taken us away from the vision of Thomas Jefferson with its stable communities and tangible connection to the country. Professor Berry dwells on our obsession for efficiency that has come to mean cheapness at any price. He dwells on our obsession for specialization that has wrought both social and ecological destruction. I quote him again: "Nowhere are these tendencies more apparent than in agriculture. For years now the agricultural specialists have tended to think and work in terms of a whole and coherent system that would maintain the fertility and the ecological health of the land over a period of centuries. . . . Ignoring the ample evidence that a healthy agriculture is highly diversified, using the greatest possible variety of animals and plants, and that it returns all organic wastes to the soil, the specialists of the laboratories have promoted the specialization of the farms, encouraging one-crop agriculture and the replacement of humus by chemicals. . . . Ignoring the considerable historical evidence that to have a productive agriculture over a long period of time, it is necessary to have a stable and prosperous rural population closely bound in sympathy and association to the land, the specialists have either connived in the dispossession of small farmers by machinery and technology, or have actively encouraged their migration into the cities."

What is perhaps saddest of all is that this perversion of agriculture has probably come about from what starts out to be the noblest of motives—the best and most food at the cheapest price. With such motives, the egg industry has been revolutionized. And so has the beef industry. And so has every single crop. But has the Maine potato farmer been helped? Or the Wisconsin dairyman? Or the New Jersey egg farmer? Or the California truck gardener? Undoubtedly some have been helped—the relatively few who

have survived, perhaps. But isn't it time to begin new policies—new programs that will specifically aid small farmers?
I think so!

For years, we as publishers have reported on developments in organic agriculture. We have in a modest sense
acted as a kind of extension service for organic growing
methods, relaying information. But the need now is too
great and the hardships too severe to continue as we have in
the past—hoping for a recommendation here and a bit of
advice there. We believe it is time for the land grant colleges
to give organic agriculture all the positive help they can.

It is time to stop playing games—to dismiss as insignifi-
cant alternatives that are already helping black share-
croppers in Virginia and Georgia to earn a decent profit by
supplying organically-grown cucumbers to urban markets.
It is time to make the most of such alternatives—and stop
treating a genuine consumer demand for quality foods as
fraudulent—or a genuine back-to-the-land movement by
people of all ages as merely a fad.

A good example of what's happening is the reported
increase in the number of students applying for admission
at two major agricultural colleges, the College of Agriculture and Life Sciences at Cornell and the State University
College of Forestry at Syracuse, New York. Said Leonard
Feddema, director of admissions at Cornell's College of
Agriculture, "We see a strong desire to get back to the earth
and treat Mother Nature with respect, as well as a great
interest in organic farming."

Edward E. Palmer, president of Syracuse's Forestry
College added, "In our admissions counseling work, we have
found nearly all the applicants deeply committed to helping
solve environmental problems. Applications for the Forestry
College in 1972 jumped 70 percent over last year, while at
Cornell's College of Agriculture, 2,610 requests for admission were recorded, compared with 2,014 last year.

Mr. Feddema said that the rise in applications started
about three years ago. High school graduates are expressing
a very strong interest in farming and biological sciences, an
interest which Feddema does not think is merely a fad.
"I don't think the student concern with ecology will fade,"
he pointed out. "They want to make contributions. They
talk with a semi-religious favor, they have a psychological

approach to country living, they want to get other people to cooperate. I feel the drive will be sustained."

What must the American people do to convince land grant colleges and the Department of Agriculture that their goals are not satisfied by continued all-out drives for "efficiency and specialization?"

CHAPTER VII

THE ADVERSARY SYSTEM IN SCIENCE EDUCATION

"In short, what is needed is a group of competent scientists who would criticize any new application of science or expansion of technology. Or more succinctly, a group of scientists who would oppose the creation of new forms of garbage while advocating means of disposing of the presently accumulated garbage. It must seem that we are suggesting an end to technological progress. Quite the contrary, we are only suggesting that technology should no longer be an end unto itself, but it should be the means by which society meets its ends."

One way to help bring environmental and survival matters into the open is through the Adversary System of Scientific Inquiry.

Around the country, the mavericks are surfacing. There's no reason to be pessimistic about their existence. Ralph Nader has shown how many qualified persons want to engage in public interest law. The same spirit exists in the sciences, and only needs a variety of opportunities to express itself—to surface in the name of environmental action.

Edward J. Vander Velde, an instructor in geography at the State University of New York in Binghamton, has been experimenting with new and different teaching techniques for several years.

While at Michigan State University in East Lansing, Vander Velde and Dr. Ronald J. Horvath developed a course that dealt specifically with field research methods and techniques in geography. They decided to "teach" the usual methods and techniques, "but *within the context* of the crisis in our ecosystem and the need to develop alternative environmental uses for human survival." Students were invited to identify a number of researchable problems in the area, and one group formed around organic agriculture and gardening.

This "eco-agriculture research group" focused upon three areas for research and action:

(1) What books, courses, texts were available at Michigan State dealing with organic methods (a bibliography of reference material and list of courses of interest to organic growers were produced—survey showed no significant research in organic agriculture at MSU farm).

(2) Land and production—50-acre site will be used this spring for garden plots by students; research group made field map of land for soil and slope characteristics.

(3) Organic farmer survey in Michigan. Forms were distributed to presidents of organic gardening clubs and organic farmers. Objective is to produce a series of maps of organic gardening and farming in Michigan which will lead to a campaign to get MSU to initiate research into organic methods. The maps will also be given to organic clubs and other ecology-action organizations.

Mr. Vander Velde reported that the desire to achieve objectives continued beyond the fall academic term, and so the student group formed AHMOAB. These letters stand for the Albert Howard Memorial Organic Agriculture Brigade.

AHMOAB has organized a special course in organic gardening principles and methods which was offered in the student-run Free University during the winter term, open to everyone in the East Lansing/MSU community. Instructors included "folk faculty." A number of organic farmers have been asked to teach specific topics/skills.

Mr. Vander Velde said: "This research group participated in an exhilarating teaching/learning experience. More importantly, it was a beginning of what promises to be a significant continuing movement in both organic education and organic agriculture."

A POSSIBLE ROLE FOR ADVERSARY CENTERS

When the state of Ohio sued Dow and Wyandotte chemical corporations for polluting Lake Erie with mercury, the case hustled on its way to the Supreme Court.

But the high court dismissed the case. It's important

to know that the Supreme Court rules only on any constitutional issues that might be present in a case. But the dismissal in this instance was based on the court's admission of scientific ignorance. Justice Harlan, writing the majority opinion, said, ". . . the scientific conclusion that mercury is a serious water pollutant is a novel one . . . whether and to what extent the existence of mercury in natural waters can safely or reasonably be tolerated is a question for which there is presently no firm answer . . . the notion that judges, even with the assistance of a most competent Special Master (a qualified expert), might appropriately undertake at this time to unravel these complexities is, to say the least, unrealistic."

Justice Douglas wrote the only dissenting opinion, and it was brilliant. He said, "The problem, though clothed in chemical secrecies, can be exposed by the experts." He cited previous cases, extremely complex, in which Special Masters helped the court through the scientific intricacies. There is also the long-held tenet propounded by Justice Holmes that allows the court to act when there is a "clear and present danger" to the welfare of the citizens of the United States.

The whole question of pollution, and the continuing discharge of toxic materials into the environment in the face of obvious evidence as to its detrimental effects, is fraught with constitutional issues. Beside the "clear and present danger" rule, the court has many times considered cases involving threats to life and property by irresponsible individuals and corporations. Precedent for legally stopping pollution *now* would not be hard to find.

But the court abdicates its responsibility by saying, "We haven't been admitted to the secret room of scientific knowledge. We can't understand." And without even trying to understand.

Enter the Adversary Center for Scientific Inquiry. Lawyers for the polluters would represent one side of the issue, representatives for the adversary center would represent the other side. From these two presentations, the court would have the scientific claims and counterclaims laid out. These can then be applied to the constitution to see if they fit. The court's responsibility is still to interpret the constitutional issues, but the pros and cons of scientific issues would be spelled out in understandable terms.

If the court tries to find Special Masters, they would have to find men who understand both pros and cons, understand the scientific issues involved, and are absolutely unbiased. Good luck. We doubt if more than a handful of such men exist, if any at all. In these days, you either see the need for an end to pollution now or later.

However, the adversary center people would more likely be fair, since they would have no vested interest in the production of the goods which cause the pollution. They would represent not only the people's side of the issue, but the unbiased scientific facts. The court could rely with assurance on the advice of a properly constituted adversary center, beholden to no one, which critically analyses the issues and isn't afraid to ask the painful questions.

Courts should back the creation of adversary centers of scientific inquiry. There is no time left for the court to wash its hands in ignorance while the citizens of this country are sickened to enrich a group of corporations.

IF SEARS CAN DO IT, WHY CAN'T THE U.S.A.?

Sears Roebuck seems to be an excellent example of product development. By a well-planned and well-implemented program, Sears manages to create new models and products which invariably bring it high ratings from such objective evaluators as *Consumer Reports*.

If the nation had such capabilities and facilities, using environmental specifications, it seems fair to assume that effective results would be achieved. The American public is no longer willing to allow only commercialism to dictate efficiency in product development. It's ridiculous to have millions and millions of dollars go into a new flavor for a soft drink or fender design, and then to have no money whatsoever to help produce a new energy source of fantastic import to the future of mankind.

The big "crunch" issue confronting anti-pollution programs now, according to Sen. Nelson's legislative director John Heritage, is employment. "You're throwing people out of work. . . . You're eliminating jobs." That's the big cry that the promoters of a particular practice in a particular industry throw out, and it puts anyone pushing an environmental cause far, far up the wall.

Certainly in some cases anti-pollution standards could

make it rough on a marginal company in a tough economic bind. But just as certain is that company executives know what a "sure thing" they have going when they scream "No jobs!" and that they're shouting that phrase before they've investigated the situation.

Take the case of strip mining. There have been many bills before the Congress to ban strip mining. The sponsors of the bills realize that it's no longer possible to try to improve strip-mining practices when such practices destroy the land so it can never be reclaimed. The coal companies and promoters of strip mining say that such legislation will put even more people in Appalachia out of work. So the sponsors of the bills face almost impossible opposition. Both labor and management fight them.

But stop for a minute and consider what an Adversary approach to strip mining might be. It might force these questions to be asked of the other side:

(1) How many jobs will be created?
     For how long?
(2) What will be the pay scales?
(3) How will the life of those workers and their families who live in the area be affected by strip mining?

An Adversary approach could conceivably show that the area now being considered for strip mining would be more worthwhile to industry, in the way of profits, and to the people, in the way of jobs, by showing how it could be used to process and recycle solid wastes which now plague urban centers in the area. In other words, an Adversary approach would have a positive, creative impact on the economy which would ultimately help industry. And it would actually provide *more and better* jobs!

It is absolutely ridiculous (and in Dr. John Gofman's words, "schizophrenic") to willingly and knowingly go into a technique like strip mining, knowing its temporary . . . destructive . . . and must be stopped, just because an industry or company (and the people temporarily benefitted with jobs) have the financial interest and ability to do so. After a relatively brief period, those jobs won't exist any more, and the company will have to go someplace else and start all over.

Adversary Centers will make it respectable for adversaries to "do their thing" without being chastised in a multitude of ways. Here we are, asking people to sacrifice themselves in a cause that means survival. And right now, adversaries face unrelenting criticism as they succeed in getting their adversary message across. The greater their effect, the harsher the criticism of their professional stature.

Adversary Centers could show industries that they can make a profit on products that won't create an ever-mounting hazard to the environment. The centers could stimulate industries in a direction that will get them to relate and communicate with the market they'll be serving in 10 years —The Young!

In our local paper recently were the names of the National Merit Scholarship winners. Two of them belong to our area environmental action groups. These young people don't want to go along with product choices and job challenges as they are. Life styles will be different, and industry will want to make products compatible with those life styles. Those youths are going to be the market—both the consumer and job market—but how will industry know what they want?

THE IDEA THAT LAUNCHED THE ADVERSARY CONCEPT

This is the original "Proposal to Establish an Adversary System of Scientific Inquiry" by Dr. John W. Gofman and Dr. Arthur R. Tamplin.

There are many things wrong with science in this country, but its major fault is that it has become a meaningless set of WPA projects. There are also many things wrong with technology in the country, but its major fault is that it does not respond to the needs of society. The present growing environmental crisis demonstrates that science and technology have actually begun to operate to the detriment of society in an obvious manner. Yet we find that the scientific advisor to the President is chosen because he supports the ABM development and that the President announces a new goal for the space program which is nothing more than a meaningless WPA project. The SST promises to be a disastrous WPA project. Then the President decides to cut the budget for the NIH, and on one can really argue that this cut will have any significant effect on medical science. The AEC pushes high energy physics and builds BEV accelerators. This is the area where the money is, so young physicists go into this area. Now the JCAE is disenchanted and the young physicists are out on a limb. In reality, there is reason to believe that the BEV program is another overrated program that grew all out of proportion.

Scientists pursuing these meaningless WPA projects do not represent a direct detriment to society. They, however, do pose an indirect threat to society in that they are used to support the concept of the omniscience and omnipotence of science and technology. They offer credibility to the proposed ABM system and thereby offer thinkability to a nuclear war; they create the illusion that if we really get into trouble with our environment, science and technology will be able to rescue us; and they divert the scientific manpower away from more meaningful programs.

Science in itself is not bad or good; that is why it has no ethics. Without application, science is meaningless. But most of science in this country is meant to be applied and, hence, the government, hand in glove with industry, rules over science by controlling the purse strings. As a consequence, science in this country must either be irrelevant or part of some mission prescribed by government in consort with industry.

Many scientists have spoken out against the ABM system, war-related research, the SST and NASA. Many have complained about the wrong priorities in mission related research. Many have sounded the alarm concerning the impending environmental crisis. Why haven't they been more effective? One reason is that the majority of scientists are "hacks" who support the proposed projects, either openly or by silence. The public, therefore, assumes that the majority of the concerned and competent scientific community supports the programs while a few dissidents are making noise. But the major reason is that it takes money and time to fight city hall. The proponents are well organized and well funded by government and industry; not so for the opponents. Moreover, the opponents must present a much stronger case against a program than the proponents present for the program.

Quite obviously we need a mechanism for effectively criticizing present day science and technology, and for articulating a new set of priorities that would lead science and technology to fulfilling the needs of society. In order to accomplish this, a group of scientists have to be funded for this purpose. Moreover, it is absolutely essential that they be funded in such a manner as to be completely independent of government and industry.

The scientists who compose this group must be activists in the best sense of the word. They must interact with members of Congress and the various activists and pressure groups in the country. The association with activists, pressure groups, and with Congress can serve two purposes. First, it will aid the scientists in understanding and articulating the basic needs of society. This will aid the groups and Congress in such articulation. Second, it will give the scientists a mechanism for creating public awareness. The one essential ingredient in this interaction is that the science be unassailable. For if the technical detail of the science is not superb, the impact will be minimal.

Their immediate role must be to undermine the unwarranted public and Congressional confidence in existing science and technology. They must show that science and technology are not meeting the needs of society and, in fact, are actually compounding the problems of society. But, at the same time, they should not be just destructive in their criticism. They must offer alternative programs that represent routes to the solution of the needs of society.

We would propose that, at most, only 100 scientists would be required. The entire program would thus cost less than five million dollars a year. These scientists would work in centers. Each center would have 10 to 15 scientists. The numbers are not arbitrary; they represent a critical and limiting mass of interacting scientists within a center, and the same applies to the number of centers.

The program would start with one such center, and the number and nature of the additional centers would evolve from the initial center's study in six months to one year. The first center would be required to structure the problem; that is, to create the framework upon which the needs of society can be related to existing science and technology. By this process they would identify the major facets of the problem, and this identification would lead to the number and nature of the other centers.

This structuring and ordering of the problem has to remain open. The first cult will probably have to be modified in many of its details. At the same time, it will be the very important first step.

Moreover, this structuring cannot be done in the abstract. It must be approached as a problem oriented project. We would suggest that this initial problem be the three faces of the GNP: gross national product, gross national power, and gross national pollution. All of these are interrelated, and the three together eventually must become self-limiting. By the year 2000 the United States population is expected to reach 300-million. An important parallel study would be to freeze the GNP at the present level and to look at the nature of technology in the year 2000 under this constraint.

It seems quite evident that science and technology have become uncoupled from our society.

In short, what is needed is a group of competent scientists who would criticize any new application of science or expansion of technology. Or more succinctly, a group of scientists who would oppose the creation of new forms of garbage while advocating means of disposing of the presently accumulated garbage. It must seem that we are suggesting an end to technological progress. Quite the contrary, we are only suggesting that technology should no longer be an end unto itself, but it should be the means by which society meets its ends.

THE NEED FOR AN ADVERSARY SYSTEM

Jerome Goldstein

In my mail recently, I received a form letter from the president of the local electric company telling how lucky I am that nuclear power was developed "just in the nick of time." In a calm, reassuring manner, he told me to ignore the few "emotional" scientists who warned about radiation dangers and nuclear accidents.

The other day, in a California farm paper, I read an article about "judicious use of fertilizer." The author is an executive with a huge petro-chemical firm that makes artificial fertilizer.

Last night, I came across a two-page advertisement in a national magazine claiming that the Alaska pipeline was nothing to worry about. It explained in detail how the ice-rich permafrost would not be hurt.

The American public, I believe, at this point in time, is being treated most unfairly. At a time when they are asking *hard* questions, they are being given soft and reassuring words.

"Don't worry" is what the big companies and the "experts" tell us. "We can give you all the cars, all the electricity, all the food, all the pleasures because

". . . we've developed safe, cheap nuclear power in the nick of time;

". . . we've developed safe, cheap pesticides in the nick of time;

". . . we've developed safe, cheap gasoline to drive more cars on safe, cheap superhighways;"

. . . and on and on with "nick-of-time" solutions ranging from the SST to miracle food additives that are supposed to "taste better than the real thing."

John Gofman and Arthur Tamplin are two scientists who are doing everything they can to develop an Adversary System of Scientific Inquiry. The University of California scientists put it this way:

> We must develop a way to develop centers of technological assessment, with the sole purpose of learning and communicating to the public the *adverse* features of technological approaches. The goal is *not* destructive criticism, but rather the full development of "the other side of the picture."

Drs. Gofman and Tamplin are living examples of the adversary idea. Both men, while working for the Atomic Energy Commission at the Lawrence Radiation Laboratory of the University of California, came up with research showing that nuclear power plants are possibly the worst environmental hazard ever created by technology. They are being asked to speak by citizen groups around the country where nuclear plants are proposed (the number of plants is expected to go from 15 to more than 500 in the next 3 decades). These citizens are tremendously worried by the dangers of radioactivity, increased infant mortality, genetic defects as well as thermal pollution.

In reply to their fears, spokesmen for the electric companies say something like this in well-modulated, computer-like style:

"There's really nothing to worry about. The best scientists in the country—in universities, in industry, and in the Atomic Energy Commission—assure us that there is no evidence of radiation side effects. We live here too, so we wouldn't expose ourselves to such dangers, would we?

"Nuclear energy has been discovered just in the nick of time. In fact, our present fossil fuel plants—those terrible coal-burning plants—are causing much more disease and death than nuclear plants will ever cause. The critic(s) who warn against nuclear power stand(s) alone. You can trust us!"

The critics of atomic power do unfortunately stand alone—in the sense that they are outnumbered to a fantastic degree. But that's what environmental protection is all about now. How do we give greater emphasis to the critics who want to save what's left, knowing full well that those critics would not win if victory depended only upon a show of hands?

And that's why Scientific Adversary Centers are so essential. We need them to make sure the right questions are asked. Only after the right questions are asked, will we get the right environmental answers!

In the field of energy, "adversary questions" would involve total power requirements for a region—what effect will it have on population and living conditions; how could present plants be cleaned up; what are the reserves of coal, gas, etc.; what are the costs of clean coal power?

After the questions come the need for adversary-type answers—not to be done by scientists connected with the industry or government agencies responsible for new power sources. Says Dr. Gofman: "At every opportunity, learn how to ask the embarrassing questions that the technologists-industrialists so bravely sweep under the rug. Confront them at every level—local, state, and national, and require that they answer the *unanswered,* if not unanswerable, questions about their proposed technologies."

What Drs. Gofman and Tamplin really want to create is a better "climate for scientific mavericks."

CHAPTER VIII

THE STUDENT AS ENVIRONMENTAL ACTIVIST

"The young people are taking up the banners of environmental protection. After all, they are the ones who are going to have to live in this horrible mess we are now making; they are going to have to wear the gas masks and struggle through the junk, and try to drink the filthy, unsafe water."

—Professor Robert Rienow,
Co-author, *Moment in the Sun*

All over the country, students are spearheading the drive for a cleaner, and more healthful environment. The movement has taken hold with phenomenal speed and strength; from a relative unknown, it has blossomed into a national cause over the past three years. Ecology, once a word heard only in biology class, now dots the newspapers daily and has become, in effect, a household term.

Eco-activists come in all shapes, sizes, colors and political affiliations; their methods range from establishment of recycling centers to the more "subversive" execution of acts of ecotage such as those committed by the legendary Fox of Kane County, Illinois. (The Fox was noted for such tactics as dumping filth from a polluted river on the rug in the reception office of the polluter, or cementing closed discharge pipes from offending plants.)

But the basic good of environmental activism is always present: that all these forces, regardless of their philosophy or intensity, are united to help make man aware of his dependence on the earth, and the earth's dependence on man's wise use of its resources.

It is now common to see students collecting their paper waste, their non-returnable bottles and cans in dormitory rooms to await a weekly collection. It is common to see them spending some of their spare time tilling a plot in a community organic garden. It is common to see them band-ing together into food co-ops or conspiracies to buy better foods. It is common to see them publishing newsletters to inform other students of environmental problems on campus and encouraging action for their correction.

An even more encouraging trend in the past few years is the newer tendency for students to branch out in their environmental activities, into the surrounding community. Often, it is effort by students alone that establishes a neighborhood recycling facility or a community organic garden, and raises the "earth consciousness" of the public-at-large. The students of the University of Michigan at Ann Arbor are an excellent example, discussed in chapter 3.

And there are others. In Oregon, the Student Public Interest Research Group reacted to industry opposition to a new law requiring deposits on beer bottles by encouraging a boycott of the brands. At Harvard, student response brought about the dropping of plastic disposable cups from the major dining hall. Students at Yale and other colleges across the country have encouraged the serving of better foods in their cafeterias, and the food services have responded.

At the School of the Ozarks, students are helping to rebuild an old water-wheel driven flour mill. Project sponsors hope it will become a student industry, grinding carefully selected grains that have been grown organically on School of the Ozarks land.

And many students have no qualms about taking on the government. At Columbia, four law students joined in petitioning the Federal Trade Commission to take action against two paper manufacturers who, they charged, failed to comply with pollution control regulations and were causing more environmental problems than most. Students Challenging Regulatory Agency Procedures (SCRAP), also petitioning the government, joined with the National Parks and Conservation Association to ask the Interstate Commerce Commission to reconsider its fixing of prices for transport of scrap materials at more than twice the rate for raw materials. Throughout this book can be found examples of students who, working together and with members of their communities, have helped to make people more aware and have helped to make the planet a little more viable.

The lines that previously separated the college campus from the community—at least where the environment is concerned—are disappearing. The scope of campus-initiated action is not just the campus; in many cases it is the neighborhood, the city, the state, the country or the world.

ECOLOGY CENTERS

To help broaden the environmental movement into the community, youthful eco-activists from around the nation met at Washington University in St. Louis late in 1970 and established a national network of ecology centers—incorporated, nonprofit, community-based organizations designed to educate and involve the community in local environmental problems. They provide ready access to basic scientific information necessary to increase public awareness and channel it into effective programs for environmental change. Some centers have set up large-scale recycling projects; many conduct seminars and teach-ins on natural foods and ecological living, provide a speakers' bureau service, run action-switchboards, and more.

The coordinating organization is the Ecology Center Communications Council Inc., which publishes a newsletter, acts as a liaison between centers and other groups or agencies, coordinates environmental projects, provides information that local centers may not have and, basically, helps things run smoothly for ecology centers all over the nation.

The ECCC also publishes an informational packet for people wishing to establish a center in their area; just write them at P.O. Box 21072, Washington, D.C. 20009.

The following list contains all the ecology centers in the U.S. and Canada that were active or developing as of mid-1972:

Pratt Remmel
Arkansas Ecology Center
316 Chester Street
Little Rock, Ark. 72201
  (501) 374-6271

Mary Taylor
Eco-Center
1424 Pearl, #7
Boulder, Colorado 80302
  (303) 447-0513

Bruce Rector
Ecology Action of
  the San Fernando Valley
9520 Etawanda
Northridge, Calif. 91324
  (213) 886-7306

Jim Jacobson
Ecology Center
Box 16177
San Diego, Calif. 92116
  (714) 583-5369

Paul Relis
Community Ecology Center
15 West Anapamu Street
Santa Barbara, Calif. 93104
  (805) 962-2210

Gil Tortolani
Monterey Ecology Center
P.O. Box 711
Pacific Grove, Calif. 93950
  (408) 372-9478

Claire Dedrick
Peninsula Conservation
  Center
885 Oak Grove
Menlo Park, Calif. 94025
  (415) 322-6671

Gil Bailie
San Francisco Ecology Center
13 Columbus Avenue
San Francisco, Calif. 94111
  (415) 391-6307

Ted Radke
Eco-Info, Inc.
834 Carquinez Way
Martinez, Calif. 94543
  (415) 937-0209

Valley Ecology Center
401 South K Street
Livermore, Calif. 94550
  (415) 443-5483

Carol Tickner
San Leandro Ecology Center
1190 Davis
San Leandro, Calif. 94577
  (415) 635-8200

South County Ecology Center
3667 Castro Valley Blvd.
Casto Valley, Calif. 94578
  (415) 582-7664

Dan DeGrassi
Berkeley Ecology Center
2179 Allston Way
Berkeley, Calif. 94704
  (415) 548-2220

Pat Heffernan
Marin Ecology Center
Box 725
San Anselmo, Calif. 94960
  (415) 383-4226

Cliff Humphrey
Ecology Action Educational
  Institute
Box 3895
Modesto, Calif. 95352
  (209) 529-3784

Charles Hinkle
Sonoma County Environ-
  mental Center
211 Santa Rosa Ave.
Santa Rosa, Calif. 95404
  (704) 545-2196

Wesley Chesboro
Northcoast Environmental
  Center
640 10th Street
Arcata, Calif. 95521
  (707) 822-6918

Curtis Meckemson
Ecology Information Center
1221 20th Street
Sacramento, Calif. 95821
  (916) 444-3174

Steve Burdick
Environment Northwest
Box 15309 Wedgewood
  Station
Seattle, Washington 98115
  (206) EM 3-4088

Robert Ascah
Environmental Pollution
    Information Center
4030 Old Orchard Road
Montreal, 260, P.Q. Canada
    (514) 484-2145

Jane McGregor
Calgary Eco-Centre
247-803 1st St. SE
Calgary, Alberta, Canada
    (403) 263-6106

CONTACTS FOR DEVELOPING CENTERS

Pat McCabe
Ecology Center of Delaware
c/o Delaware League for
    Planned Parenthood
825 Washington Ave.
Wilmington, Delaware 19801
    (302) 652-3948

Mr. Joe C. Matthews
Government Center
Winston-Salem, N.C. 27101
    (919) 727-2071

Bill Rosen
EEO Reading Room
101 Lefevre Hall
University of Missouri
Columbia, Missouri 65201

Nancy Pearlman
Ecology Representative
P.O. Box 24388
Los Angeles, Calif. 90024

Harry Wyeth
Solano Ecology Center
P.O. Box 991
Fairfield, Calif. 94533
    (707) 425-6225

Happy Nelson
Vermont Environment Center
Ripton, Vermont 05766
    (802) 388-7833

Melville Thomason
New Canaan Nature Center
144 Oenoke Ridge
New Canaan, Conn. 06840
    (203) 966-9577

Monmouth Eco-Center
629 Mattison Ave.
Asbury Park, N.J. 07712
    (201) 775-4949

Tom Stokes
Enviromental Mobilization
    Fund
549 W. 52nd Street
New York, New York 10019
    (212) 581-0127

Carl Simons
Philadelphia Ecology Action
    Group
3907 Spruce St.
Philadelphia, Pa. 19104
    (215) BA 2-5247

William Painter
Washington Ecology Center
2000 P St., NW
Washington, D.C. 20036
    (202) 833-1778

Barbara Swaczey
Ecology Action Center
112 East 25th St.
Baltimore, Md. 21218
    (301) 366-2070

Robbie Ellyson
Richmond Ecology Center
2315 Monument Avenue
Richmond, Va. 23220
    (703) 355-4391

Barbara Irvine
Environmental Information
    Center
P.O. Box 922
Sarasota, Fla. 33578
    (813) 355-6967

Alan Sandler
Tampa Bay Ecology Center
6739 Elm Court
Tampa, Fla. 33602
(813) 238-5163

Dan Zilko
Canton Ecology Center
218 6th Street, NW
Canton, Ohio 44702
(216) 454-9941

Mike Schectman
Ecology Center of Ann Arbor
417 Detroit
Ann Arbor, Mich. 48104
(313) 761-3186

Sue Denig
Environmental Headquarters
310 S. Blackstone
Jackson, Michigan 49201
(517) 783-1879

Joan Minczeski
Midwest Environmental
  Education and Research
  Assoc. (MEERA)
295 Summit Ave.
St. Paul, Minn. 55102
(612) 222-3350

Wes George
North Shore Ecology Center
747 Central
Highland Park, Ill. 60035
(312) 432-1440

Stuart Liederman
Environmental Response
Box 1124
Washington University
St. Louis, Missouri 63130
(314) 863-0100 Ext. 4070

Ross Vincent
Ecology Center of Louisiana
Box 15149
New Orleans, La. 70115
(504) 522-4008

Still other student eco-activists are going past community affairs and entering the national environmental scene, on both government and industrial levels. They are attempting to convince their school administrations to vote stock proxies with an acute awareness of the environmental effects of their holdings. Senator Lee Metcalf (D.-Mont.) has voiced his support of this type of action, and even encouraged it, to bring about "Changes in public policy which are beyond the reach of public officials."

"No one," he added, "has ever determined the potential which universities have for influencing corporate policy through voting of common stock. It is my firm belief that the faculties, students, administration and alumni of our great universities could perform monumental services to their country at a critical point in its history by redirection of the voting power of university stock in energy corporations.

"This academic exercise would also be invaluable in impressing upon those who undertook it the fact that no one knows who owns America, and that corporate reporting requirements are grossly inadequate."

Sen. Metcalf began looking into the situation, he said, because "the practices and policies of energy companies, more than any other segment of our society, lead to concern over environmental protection, health and safety, equal employment opportunity, economic concentration and over-pricing."

With 53 of the country's major universities holding over 11 million shares of stock in 44 oil companies, over 10 million shares of stock in 85 electric utilities and over 1 million shares of stock in gas utilities, the possibilities for academic influence over energy policies are open. Students are just beginning to realize this potential, and are beginning drives at many universities to try to influence these policies in an environmentally positive way.

FOR THE FUTURE

Student activism, however, cannot do the whole job. And it is likely that people who are interested in environmental studies will, eventually, be interested in environmental careers. Until recently, however, there has been a dearth of guidance information in that field.

Odom Fanning, a science writer whose personal and professional interest in environmental protection has spanned more than 20 years, has written a book entitled *Opportunities in Environmental Careers*. Fanning, a special assistant for technical information in the U.S. Commerce Department, has been an editor, columnist and writer for private, government and service organizations, and was editor-in-chief of the First Annual Report on Environmental Quality for the President's Council on Environmental Quality in 1970.

Unlike the Report, this current work is a personal effort, reflecting his own analyses, opinions and projections about the need for environmental specialists, and is backed up by an impressive amount of factual materials.

Starting with a brief review of early environmental concern by few, and the later, recent recognition of a crisis by many, he quickly relates what has been done to make elementary and high school age youths aware of the environment in which they live. The emphasis here, as it is throughout the book, is on what similar activities can continue to be done—and improved upon—in the light of what has already been learned.

With little delay, he moves into the subject of environmental management, the term which encompasses the remaining subject matter of the book. As he puts it, *"Environmental management* seems to be a well-accepted general term to embrace all activities, public and private, undertaken to achieve the goal of environmental quality."

Then, using a classification system devised by the U.S. Senate, and reproduced in the book, he breaks down the *activities* of environmental management into five categories, each of which contains a varying number of subcategories useful to any person approaching the study of the environment.

From there, he jumps into another breakdown of environmental management, this one according to five major fields—ecology, earth sciences, resources and recreation, environmental design and environmental protection—which he describes as "an arbitrary classification but workable from the viewpoints of student, teacher, parent, or school administrator." He later devotes a complete chapter to each of these fields, treating them in depth.

While this book is a practical tool for any person wishing to grasp the full scope of environmental activities, it is strongly directed at the person who intends to pursue a career in one of these fields. With that in mind, Fanning presents a chart (adapted from the National Sanitation Foundation)—two vertical columns representing the Academic Ladder and the Career Ladder—enabling the reader to visually comprehend the jobs available to various academic levels, ranging from the high school dropout to the doctorate of science or engineering.

This done, he presents sample curricula for a two year environmental technician as well as a four year engineering student. Such right-to-the-point information, in the form of the charts or tables, and in the text as well are what make this book the practical guide that it is.

And it doesn't stop there.

In fact, you might as well pick up some postage stamps before you read Fanning's book, for a sizable portion of the information that he shares with his readers has not been predigested. Most chapter endings carry listings of organizations and their available literature which you can obtain if you want to investigate and evaluate environmental careers and activities. You will find 51—count them—such items listed, some free, others which cost.

He rounds out the book with six appendices which contain, in order: a bibliography of inexpensive books about the environment; a list of periodicals covering the environment; voluntary organizations open to public membership; key government agencies in environmental management; institutions offering training in environmental technology; and finally a listing of one hundred leading university environmental science centers, which includes the names of both the institutions and the programs, their operational objectives, and the scholastic scope, requirements and enrollment (when that information is available).

While Fanning's book is of great value for those who plan professional careers in environmental management, it is also an excellent guide for full or part time ecological activists and contains a collection of titles that represent countless hours of environmental reading for any person wishing to learn more about the world which surrounds him.

Opportunities in Environmental Careers is published by Vocational Guidance Manuals (the educational books division of Universal Publishing and Distributing Corporation) 235 E. 45th St., New York, N.Y. 10017. ($5.75)

SOURCES OF ENVIRONMENTAL-ORGANIC EDUCATION

What do you want incoming freshmen to know when they arrive in your first-year course?

(1) I want them to know that life is exciting, full of mystery, challenging—to sense that life is a give-and-take love affair with the environment, for better or for worse. And that death is a normal and desirable end.

(2) I'd like them to have cared for an animal in captivity, to have worried about its welfare, and to have been truly responsible; and similarly to have cared for a captive plant for a year or more.

(3) I would wish they had all had a plot of ground outdoors, not necessarily circumscribed and called a garden, to wonder over and to work over for three seasons.

(4) I would like to have had them teach a young child about life, and as a result to have their own questioning deepened.

(5) If they can run a soil test, band a bird, prune a tree—good. If they can enjoy looking through a microscope for two hours because they can handle it effectively—fine. If they know the periodic table and can climb the spiral DNA—excellent. But these things are unimportant compared to items one through four.

—"A Nature Study Viewpoint"
Dr. John W. Brainaerd
Springfield College
Springfield, Massachusetts

CHAPTER IX

CLASSROOMS FOR ORGANIC LIVING

Classrooms everywhere are going organic. Courses, workshops, seminars, lectures, independent-study programs —educators are seeking ways to channel the tide of organic-learning ambition into the system. Right from kindergarten through a dozen grades of public school, on up to collegiate, post-grad, community-group and even senior-citizen level, the call for organic-living know-how is creating change.

Right now more than 7,000 New Jersey elementary school children are learning all about organic gardening, preparing healthful organic food snacks in their classrooms, and even having fun with a new type of exercise program designed to aid heart health. It's part of a new organic educational services program developed by Rodale Press in cooperation with New Jersey's Technology for Children Project.

T 4 C, as it is called, is a special learn-by-doing inter-disciplinary approach to education covering the area of social studies, science, math and language arts. About a year ago the project directors wrote us: "We are interested in any curriculum materials dealing with environmental education that would be appropriate for grades K-6. If you can suggest any courses of study covering the numerous problems that are facing us today, it would be of tremendous assistance to our teachers in Project Technology for Children, which numbers several hundred—involving thousands of school children."

Organic Gardening and Farming, Prevention and Fitness For Living editors went to work. We prepared special materials and teaching aids and were asked to conduct a two-week workshop for Technology for Children supervising teachers. Through a series of more than 30 projects contained in a special kit, these teachers learned the philosophy and principles of organic living. They participated in making compost, testing soil, recycling school paper and waste, planting seeds, sprouting grains, making peanut butter, granola and other healthful snacks—even participating in a special kids' exercise session. Each teacher was given a kit containing background information on the projects so that he could pass it on to other instructors in his school district.

Today more than 143 New Jersey schools are teaching the basic principles of organic living. But Rodale Press and Technology for Children are going one step further. Cafeteria personnel in one T 4 C school are being taught how to serve and prepare organic food lunches. At another school, teachers and children will be planting an organic garden. These schools will serve as demonstration centers for teachers from all over the state to come and learn the organic living principles.

Natural Food Careers in New York City, Gardening Course in Washington High School

The Board of Education of the City of New York has a feasibility study under way to determine whether it should "introduce into the curricula of N.Y. City High Schools a course of study which would prepare students for careers in the natural food industry." That's a significant breakthrough, to say the least. Milton Rogers, the board's Project Director for Natural Food Careers, initiated his drive for the course by contacting Organic Gardening and Farming and Organic Food Marketing.

Rogers' idea centers around the conviction that organically-grown foods—and everything connected with providing them—are the coming thing. He's convinced, too, that businesses will need and want qualified workers in every phase of the trade. Based on that, his recommendations have zeroed in on the vocational opportunities in growing, distributing, marketing and preparing natural foods.

Other Elementary and High School Courses

COLLINS SCHOOL
Grand Rapids, Michigan

Science department coordinator Eugene Greer writes, "I teach four classes of sixth grade science (total of 135 students) in a suburban area. Several students have their own gardens. This year we have a class project consisting of a large garden plot and several raised planter areas. We will be using organic methods and developing a large compost heap for use on the garden and flower areas."

BROOKFIELD HIGH SCHOOL
Brookfield, Connecticut

Organic Gardening and Farming magazine reader Gustaf A. Nelson was asked to give an organic gardening course to local high school students interested in the subject as an elective. "It is something they have requested and for which they will receive no credit associated with the required subjects. There are to be two one hour classes per week for as many weeks in the semester as may be needed to be productive. Girls and boys have applied from all classes (freshman through senior)," Nelson writes.

ALMA MIDDLE SCHOOL
Alma, Michigan

Glenn Studebaker, science instructor writes, "I am presently teaching a seventh grade science course and wish to include a session on house plants and organic gardening. We plan to test soils from backyards, determine Ph and fertilizer needs of the soil. We will also construct a hot frame and plant seeds for spring gardens."

LITTLE BRITAIN ELEMENTARY SCHOOL
Newburgh, New York

Third grade teacher Debbie Moore has her students working on indoor organic gardening and composting projects.

BATTLE CREEK PUBLIC SCHOOLS
Battle Creek, Michigan

For years, third graders in the Battle Creek Public School System were involved in a non-organic gardening program, using chemical fertilizers and pest controls. This year Battle Creek is converting its district-wide third grade gardening program to organic methods of growing.

ALBION COLLEGE
Albion, Michigan

A course in Natural Farming is offered at Albion College.

The rationale for the program is based on the assumption that the contemporary student should be offered the opportunity to understand his relationship to the land.

For further information, contact:

> Joan Sapula
> Albion College
> Albion, Michigan 49224

AMBASSADOR COLLEGE
Big Sandy, Texas

At Ambassador College, an elective course in organic agriculture is part of the regular liberal arts curriculum. There's a 4,000-acre experimental farm, plus an extensive library on natural farming and livestock raising, and a well-equipped ag laboratory. Students here not only work the fields and fresh produce gardens during their two-semester study, but also feed both this campus and the Ambassador College campus at Pasadena, California. In England, at Bricket Wood, is a third Ambassador campus with a similar agricultural program on 180 acres, stressing ecology, soil conservation and natural balance.

For further information, contact:

> Ambassador College
> Big Sandy, Texas 75755

UNIVERSITY OF CALIFORNIA BERKELEY
Berkeley, California

Dr. Bargyla Rateaver teaches a course in Conservation Gardening at the University of California, Berkeley Campus. A part of the Soils and Plant Nutrition department, this course will include a large demonstration plot and a 200-square foot plot per student.

Dr. Rateaver also will be teaching this gardening course at:

U. C. San Diego, U. C. Santa Cruz (Palo Alto), San Bernadino State College, Sacramento State College and Santa Rose Junior College.

For further information, contact:

University of California, Berkeley
Berkeley, California 94720

UNIVERSITY OF CALIFORNIA SANTA CRUZ
Santa Cruz, California

The garden project at the University of California Santa Cruz was started over five years ago. While the project was at first an informal one that needed financial help from those eager to see it take hold, it has gained official status, being made a funded UC program.

For further information, contact:

University of California Santa Cruz
Santa Cruz, California 95060

MAUI'S FREE UNIVERSITY OF LIFE
Paia Island of Maui, Hawaii

This university was formed by a handful of organic people—those individuals living on organic homesteads, growing and eating organic food. Its main purpose is to provide an atmosphere and place where anyone could come and learn the principles of organic living. An old community center was donated by the county for use by the university. Courses receiving the greatest response were the

Living Naturally in Hawaii and Homemaking Techniques. For further information contact:

Mauna Olu College
Paia Island of Maui, Hawaii 96779

OTHER COURSES

The following colleges and universities reportedly have courses in organic living; however, no further information was available.

Arizona State University
Tempe, Arizona 85281

Cornell University
Ithaca, New York 14850

Fairhaven College
Bellingham, Wash. 98225

Florida Presbyterian College
St. Petersburg, Florida 33733

Hampshire College
Amherst, Mass. 01002

University of Illinois
Urbana, Illinois 61801

University of Iowa
Iowa City, Iowa 52240

Iowa State University
Ames, Iowa 50010

University of Massachusetts
Amherst, Mass. 01002

Michigan State University
East Lansing, Mich. 48823

Oregon State University
Corvallis, Oregon 97331

Pennsylvania State
University
University Park, Pa. 16802

Sacramento State College
Sacramento, Calif. 95819

Sarah Lawrence College
Bronxville, New York 10708

University of Washington
Seattle, Washington 98105

CHAPTER X

ENVIRONMENT-RELATED COURSE OFFERINGS

By now, the issue of environmental protection has progressed from an obscure cause to an integrated part of the lives of society. Offerings of colleges and universities reflect this change; courses that were once scattered among many departments or, in fact, were not offered at all have now been collected in many cases under the department heading of Environmental Studies or Environmental Sciences.

Take, for example, the prospectus for John Remsberg's three-credit course at the University of Michigan in Ann Arbor, "Living with the Earth":

PURPOSE: To introduce many "alternative life skills" useful in living in close ecological balance with the environment. The "environment" may be an organic garden, a homestead or a small community. For the purpose of giving this course a focus, we will heavily emphasize Ann Arbor's Community Organic Garden on North Campus. This seven-acre site will serve as a focal point for food (plant and animal production, storage, energy production (from sun and wind)) and total recycling of everything possible.

The following list reflects response from a large number of colleges and universities across the country; yet there are undoubtedly other courses and curricula that we have not yet uncovered. These will hopefully be included in future editions.

The listing is in alphabetical order. Institutions beginning with "University of . . ." are listed by their place name; for example, University of California is listed under

"C", as California, University of. An index by state is provided in the back of this book.

ADAMS STATE COLLEGE
Alamosa, Colorado

Adams State College offers a unique curriculum that integrates the biological, chemical, economic, geological, physical, political and psychological aspects of the environment. A rigorous, four year course of study, the program includes such topics as: Natural Resources, Introductory Atmospheric Science, Man's Influence on the Natural Environment, Population and Human Ecology, Pollution Effects, Environmental Effects on Health, Treatment of Data, Politics and Economics of Environmental Management, Methods and Techniques of Pollution Detection and Control, Ecology for Environmentalists, and Conservation.

For further information, contact:

> Dr. Richard C. Peterson
> Director of Environmental Science
> Adams State College
> Alamosa, Colorado 81101

UNIVERSITY OF ALASKA
College, Alaska

The University of Alaska has a program leading to a Bachelor of Arts in Renewable Resource Management designed for students who want to go on to graduate work in the broad resources area or for those who want a general university-level education emphasizing renewable resources and their management.

In order to assure the success of the Environmental Studies Program at the University of Alaska, the university has received a grant supporting travel to selected universities with environmental studies, allowing the university to benefit from the good and bad experiences of earlier attempts at such curricula.

In addition to the program leading to a Bachelor of Arts in Renewable Resource Management, the university also offers programs in Environmental Health Engineering and Environmental Health Science.

Recent programs include the Point Hope Research Project, an extra-curricular endeavor in which students studied the slow decay of the natural resources of the area. Through their observations, the students decided that there was not much that they could do to retard the Point Hope's slow decay. The decay stems from causes too deep to be influenced. What they could, and did, do was document the change, understand something of the old ways, and see how and why those ways fail to compete in the white man's world which is increasingly affecting even this northern outpost.

For further information, contact:

> Robert B. Weeden
> Professor of Wildlife Management
> University of Alaska
> College, Alaska 99701

THE UNIVERSITY OF ALABAMA IN BIRMINGHAM
Birmingham, Alabama
ENVIRONMENTAL SCIENCES

This environmental science major covers the topics of air and water pollution, solid wastes, land use, pesticides, radiation, energy, population growth and resources.

For further information, contact:

> University of Alabama
> Birmingham, Alabama 35233

ALFRED UNIVERSITY
Alfred, New York
ENVIRONMENTAL STUDIES

This program is designed to afford the student an opportunity to develop an expertise in a particular discipline plus a degree of familiarity with other disciplines which impinge upon some particular facet of our general environmental problem. At the same time, it enables the student to gain an appreciation of the problems of humanity and to discover those he would most like to help solve.

The graduate is especially prepared to work constructively within his own disciplines and in cooperation with environmental specialists and agencies toward mutually desirable ends.

In addition to the campus proper, facilities include terrestrial habitats on nearby University and State property and aquatic habitats of local streams, lakes, and ponds, plus the facilities of the Aquatic Institute of the College Center of the Finger Lakes at Seneca Lake.

For further information, write:

> Box 851
> Alfred University
> Alfred, New York 14802

ANDERSON COLLEGE
Anderson, Indiana

ENVIRONMENTAL SCIENCE

There is a four year Environmental Science major at Anderson College. It is interdisciplinary in nature and the recommended program includes courses in the following areas: chemistry, biology, physics, sociology, economics, psychology, philosophy, and art.

For further information, contact:

> E. G. Stedman
> Director of Environment Science
> Anderson College
> Anderson, Indiana 46012

ANNA MARIA COLLEGE
Paxton, Massachusetts

ENVIRONMENTAL HEALTH

Anna Maria College offers an interdisciplinary major in Environmental Health.

For further information, contact:

> Anna Maria College
> Paxton, Massachusetts 01612

ANTIOCH COLLEGE
Yellow Springs, Ohio

ENVIRONMENTAL STUDIES

Antioch College has comprehensive environmental studies courses involving interdisciplinary courses, seminars and workshops utilizing Glen Helen, the school's 1,000-acre outdoor laboratory.

Students can get a complete perspective on environmental problems by studying in England, Japan, Yugoslavia and other foreign countries, or in the Sonoran Desert or Southeastern seaboard, each with its own different demands on ecological balance.

For activists, there's plenty to do. Antioch is working to correct its own environmental problems and those of the local community, including air, water, soil and noise pollution. There is also an educational publication, *Environmental Leaflets,* to communicate information about the local environment to the public.

For further information, contact:

Antioch College
Yellow Springs, Ohio 45387

AUSTIN PEAY STATE UNIVERSITY
Clarksville, Tennessee

*ENVIRONMENTAL SCIENCE PROGRAM
FOR TEACHERS*

A new, multi-disciplinary environmental sciences program for teachers is being developed by the Department of Biology at Austin Peay State University. The program is based upon the urgent need for secondary science teachers who can recognize environmental patterns and processes and who can analyze and synthesize fundamental principles of social psychology, ethics and ethnology.

For further information, contact:

Department of Biology
Austin Peay State University
Clarksville, Tennessee 37040

BALL STATE UNIVERSITY
Muncie, Indiana

NATURAL RESOURCES PROGRAM

This major is multidisciplinary because the study of natural resources is a field requiring new ideas, diverse skills and integrated approaches. Students may include work from many departments in addition to a number of courses in Natural Resources which have been developed specifically for this major.

Students enrolled in the Natural Resources Program may elect a general major or specialize in such areas as resource geography, fishery resources or communications. The core requirement which all students complete includes Introduction to Natural Resources, Physical Geology, Water Resources, Soil Resources, Mineral Resources, Air Resources, Ecology, and Integrated Resources Management. The other courses elected by the student will be determined by the option selected, the student's background and his professional employment interests. In addition to the traditional science courses, others which may be included are political science, sociology, communications, physical education, statistics, computer techniques, urban and regional studies, and landscape architecture.

NATURAL RESOURCES MINOR

This is a multidisciplinary minor because the conservation of natural resources is a field of all university concern, requiring new ideas, diverse skills and integrated approaches. Students enrolled in many departments of the University, including Biology, Earth Science, Geography, Geology, Landscape Architecture, Physical Education, Regional, Urban Studies and certain areas of the Social Sciences are encouraged to elect this minor. Other students are encouraged to elect this curriculum as a "cultural" or "general education" type of minor.

BARNARD COLLEGE OF COLUMBIA UNIVERSITY
New York, New York

ENVIRONMENTAL CONSERVATION & MANAGEMENT

The goals of the program in Environmental Conservation & Management are: (1) To train and equip students with the requisite skills, values, and attitudes to enable them to participate in the work of designing, establishing, and maintaining a viable ecologic habitat for man, and (2) to promote the development of research skills in environmental science. The concept of the ecosystem lends unity to the multidisciplinary character of environmental studies.

The academic program is designed around the idea that man's ecosystem is the set of interacting relationships among the physical, biological, and cultural forces that govern the human realm. Coherence is provided by core courses followed by in-depth studies along one of several subject matter or managerial tracks.

A cluster of conservation courses on field work, readings, lab projects and internships has been developed. Students may opt to follow a managerial or a scientific program. Model programs are available from the committee. The core plus five advanced electives, one of which should be a one-year seminar, satisfy the major requirements. Examples of specialized paths are: biological conservation, environmental and physical resources, coastal zone, urban and suburban planning, and environmental center operation. Details are available from committee members.

For further information, contact:

> Leonard Zobler
> Professor of Geography
> Barnard College
> Columbia University
> New York, New York 10027

BELOIT COLLEGE
Beloit, Wisconsin

ENVIRONVAN PROGRAM

Dr. Edward Fuller, professor and Chairman of the Department of Chemistry at this small Wisconsin college, believes that "the only way that we can persuade people to make changes through political and economic processes is to make them aware of the absolute necessity of doing so."

Beloit presently is following this line of thought. Eight of its departments and programs last term offered 21 courses that dealt with the environment or had environmental emphasis. About the same number of similar courses are being offered this term.

During the winter term of 1971-72, 20 Beloit students observed results of the type of legislation, interdisciplinary seminar on environmental problems in Germany and Sweden.

All this is rather impressive, but the big thing at Beloit is their Environvan Program. This is an external environmental education program, which saw a two-man team take its Environvan into 78 high schools along the Mississippi River in the fall of 1970 and visit more than 24,000 students with a presentation on the "Ecology of the Mississippi River."

This year's program, funded by a grant from the U.S. Office of Education, will consist of five teams visiting high school students and community groups along seven bodies of water in the upper Midwest.

In addition to the Environvan Program, Beloit College also has two environmental-oriented groups on its campus. The more formal one is the Conservation Club. The other, perhaps more of a living arrangement, is Ecology House. The latter is one of a number of single-interest housing groups that the college has. A group of students rents a house from the college and literally becomes a family. Periodically the Ecology House residents will sponsor an organic dinner that is open to the public.

Conservation Club is much more public-oriented than Ecology House. Begun about three years ago, it has had its ups and downs. Its crowning hour, to this point, was the first Rock River Cleanup—the first time in modern memory that anyone endeavored to clean the Banks of the Rock River. The whole cleanup project was engineered by the students. The second year, the Club entered into a coalition with a couple of city groups for an expanded version of the cleanup—another success.

The Club keeps extensive files on environmental matters, both local and more widespread. It truly serves as an adjunct to what can be considered a good selection of environment-oriented courses in trying to make the concept of "environment" something that everyone understands, not only activists.

The Environmental Impact Committee works with the

College (as an institution) to develop ways that the College will become more operationally environment conscious.

For further information, contact:

> Richard L. Sine
> Director of Public Relations
> Beloit College
> Beloit, Wisconsin 53511
> 608/365-3391, ext. 215

BEMIDJI STATE COLLEGE
Bemidji, Minnesota
CENTER FOR ENVIRONMENTAL STUDIES

The Center for Environmental Studies is made up of members of the college faculty whose research interests involve the environment and man's relationship to his environment. The center seeks to provide facilities and resources for environmental research by undergraduate students, graduate students and faculty, often in cooperation with other schools and organizations, and to act as an educational resource on environmental topics for the people and communities of this region.

Environmental studies necessarily involve research in both the natural and the social sciences. Students will take part in environmental research in both areas, in order that they may themselves become more effective in solving human problems which relate to the environment. In addition to providing opportunities for student research, the Center is developing a special program of community-oriented research for honor students and will act as a clearing house for off-campus research and on-the-job training related to the environment.

Bemidji State College also offers programs in Fisheries and Wildlife Management.

For further information, contact:
> Mr. James P. Ludwig, Director
> Center for Environmental Studies
> Bemidji State College
> Bemidji, Minnesota 56601

BETHEL COLLEGE
North Newton, Kansas

ENVIRONMENTAL STUDIES

The Environmental Studies Program at Bethel College is planned for concerned undergraduate students who want to prepare for relevant action in the Environmental Decade and beyond. The program also prepares students for responsible citizenship no matter what profession they enter. This program offers:

(1) A multi-disciplinary understanding of environmental systems.

(2) A concern with value systems and their effect on environmental decisions.

(3) Independent student-planned research on environment problems.

(4) Flexibility in meeting requirements for many environment-related professions.

This new program will provide a major in Environmental Studies or will allow a student to broaden one of the traditional majors with a minor in Environmental Studies. The Major in Environmental Studies has four requirements:

(1) Natural Science and Mathematics—includes courses in biology, chemistry, mathematics, and earth science. The course in earth science will usually be taken at Wichita State University through a cooperative program.

(2) Social Science—includes courses in economics and population.

(3) Interdisciplinary Environment Area—includes a multi-disciplinary seminar on selected environmental topics, a seminar on value systems and environment, and an independent study program on environmental problems.

(4) Emphasis—includes additional courses in one division, either natural science or social science, to complete an emphasis in that division.

Recognizing its importance for scientific research, its historic value and its scenic beauty, Bethel College and the Nature Conservancy have acquired an 80-acre tract of land in the sandhills of south-central Kansas to be known as the

Sand Prairie Natural History Reservation. The Reservation will be used to serve many useful purposes in the study of the environment at Bethel College.

For further information, contact:

> Environmental Studies Program
> Bethel College
> North Newton, Kansas 67117

BOWLING GREEN STATE UNIVERSITY
Bowling Green, Ohio

ENVIRONMENTAL STUDIES (UNDERGRADUATE PROGRAMS)

Studies of the environment are too diverse to be encompassed by any one discipline, but no one individual can become expert across the total range of studies. Environmental Studies at Bowling Green have been designed to meet this dilemma.

Inter-disciplinary courses of study within each of the undergraduate colleges have been approved and will be fully operational by Fall 1971.

All of these programs aim at flexibility, at being able to encompass the new developments and meet the changing needs of environmental concern. This means that fundamental knowledge has been combined with an interdisciplinary view.

Because many environmental problems are practical problems, classroom work alone is inadequate for providing understanding. Consequently, internships or periods of relevant employment by government or industry are part of these programs.

ENVIRONMENTAL ADMINISTRATION MAJOR
BACHELOR OF SCIENCE IN BUSINESS
ADMINISTRATION

The importance of management and administration of environmental resources can hardly be over-estimated today. Students in this major will take advantage of the structured program of the college which will provide them with the knowledge of the behavioral, scientific, and quantitative systems associated with problems of attaining environmental quality. Students may find employment in land and urban planning offices, resource management, planning for delivery of health care, including hospital management, and at various levels of community action.

PLANNED PROGRAM
IN ENVIRONMENTAL STUDIES
BACHELOR OF SCIENCE

The student with a foundation in natural and social science can find many opportunities. The Public Health Sanitarian is involved in establishing and maintaining standards in rural and urban environments for food, water, and housing; increasingly he has been concerned with pollution monitoring and control. The Pest Control Operator, as a businessman, is an important adjunct to public officials in creating and maintaining healthful environments. Similarly, employment opportunities exist in state and federal agencies relating to wildlife, plant pest control, food and drug inspection, and other aspects of quality control.

ENVIRONMENTAL SCIENCE MAJOR
BACHELOR OF SCIENCE IN EDUCATION

The demand for health educators has always exceeded the supply, and the need for individuals to express and interpret both personal and community health as an integral part of the total environment is even more urgent now. Employment opportunities exist in health departments (health education, social work), voluntary agencies (like TB Association, Cancer Society, etc.), and industrial hygiene programs. Certification to teach general science, biology, and health in secondary schools can be obtained.

For further information, contact:

Dr. William B. Jackson
Director
Environmental Studies Center
Bowling Green State University
Bowling Green, Ohio 43403

BUCKNELL UNIVERSITY
Lewisburg, Pennsylvania

INTERDEPARTMENTAL MAJOR

At present, students wishing to pursue studies in the human environment at Bucknell are best advised to enroll in an interdepartmental major. This procedure permits a large degree of freedom in the design of the course schedule and the degree of emphasis or specialization in any given discipline.

The presence of the College of Engineering gives Bucknell considerable breadth in its approach to environmental perspectives, yet the relatively small size of the student body and low student-faculty ratio (about 13:1) allow for close personal interactions among students and between students and faculty.

The most distinctive feature of Bucknell's developing environmental program is its very close intermeshing of classroom and laboratory background with practical field and community experience, utilizing the university ecosystem and the local area as a natural laboratory. Students are encouraged to become actively involved in measuring environmental parameters and testing solutions to environmental problems.

For further information, contact:

Denis E. Marchand, Chairman
Environmental Coordinating and Advisory
  Committee
Bucknell University
Lewisburg, Pennsylvania 17837

BRANDEIS UNIVERSITY
Waltham, Massachusetts

ENVIRONMENTAL STUDIES

The Environmental Studies Program at Brandeis provides the scientific groundwork that enables individuals to consider the important social and political issues associated with the environment.

For further information, contact:

Brandeis University
Waltham, Massachusetts 02154

CALIFORNIA INSTITUTE OF TECHNOLOGY
Pasadena, California

ENVIRONMENTAL QUALITY LABORATORY

The Environmental Quality Laboratory, organized by CalTech with the cooperation of the Jet Propulsion Laboratory and the Rand Corporation, was created to deal with broad, strategic questions of environmental control. EQL consists of a small, informally organized group of strongly interacting faculty and staff members of CalTech, JPL, and Rand from various disciplines, including engineers, natural and social scientists, and systems analysts, plus several undergraduate and graduate students and post-doctoral fellows from CalTech and from the Rand summer program.

For further information, contact:

California Institute of Technology
Pasadena, California 91109

CALIFORNIA STATE COLLEGE
Dominguez Hills, California

*URBAN-ENVIRONMENTAL MANAGEMENT
PROGRAM IN URBAN STUDIES*

The Institute of Urban-Environmental Management offers inter-disciplinary programs in Urban Management and Environmental Management that lead to the Bachelor of Arts degree in Urban Studies.

The Urban-Environmental Management Programs fulfill both the departmental and interdepartmental fields of concentration requirements for the Bachelor of Arts degree at the California State College, Dominguez Hills. The programs are designed to normally extend over 12 full quarters of academic work (three quarters during each of four academic years), but progress may be accelerated through summer sessions, acceptable extension course work, or credit by examination.

For further information, contact:

California State College
Dominguez Hills, California 90246

CALIFORNIA STATE POLYTECHNIC COLLEGE
San Luis Obispo, California

ENVIRONMENTAL ENGINEERING

California State Polytechnic College has a program in Environmental Engineering.

For further information, contact:

California State Polytechnic College
San Luis Obispo, California 93401

UNIVERSITY OF CALIFORNIA AT DAVIS
Davis, California

ENVIRONMENTAL SCIENCE

This University has an undergraduate program in environmental sciences. Research facilities for modern studies on many diverse kinds of organisms, environments and resources are available. The Institute of Ecology operates an animal behavior laboratory and two limnological stations. In addition, well-equipped and staffed University stations covering a range of natural and managed ecosystems are close at hand; marine, coastal mountain, agricultural, and Sierran foothill and alpine sites are included. The library contains 750,000 volumes and its coverage in ecology is excellent.

For further information, contact:

Institute of Ecology
University of California
Davis, California 95616

UNIVERSITY OF CALIFORNIA AT IRVINE
Irvine, California

ENVIRONMENTAL SCIENCE

Another course aimed at teaching pollution fighters is being run by the University of California at Irvine. This program is retraining unemployed engineers.

For further information, contact:

University of California
Irvine, California 92664

UNIVERSITY OF CALIFORNIA AT RIVERSIDE
Riverside, California

ENVIRONMENTAL SCIENCES

Two degree options, B.S. and B.A., are offered in Environmental Sciences at this University.

For further information, contact:

John Letey, Jr.
2440 Geology Building
University of California
Riverside, California 92502

UNIVERSITY OF CALIFORNIA SANTA BARBARA
Santa Barbara, California

ENVIRONMENTAL STUDIES

This Environmental Studies major is designed to give the student a knowledge of the characteristics of the environment and the working approaches to the solution of environmental problems.

For further information, contact:

University of California
Santa Barbara, California 93106

UNIVERSITY OF CALIFORNIA, SANTA CRUZ
Santa Cruz, California

ENVIRONMENTAL STUDIES

Founded on the premise that the university should participate directly in the solution of environmental problems, the environmental studies program at the University of California, Santa Cruz, sponsors an undergraduate major that operates a central office on campus and initiates research and public service projects. As it is now, the environmental studies program is a central agency stimulating the growth of environmental concern throughout the campus, taking advantage of the Santa Cruz flexibility without treading on the toes of other existing programs. Workshops, seminars, lectures and problem-oriented task forces bring students, faculty, and non-academic professionals together in investigations of specific issues. In addition, through several seminars, students and faculty are working to develop a theoretical base for the analysis of complex environmental problems. In these projects the distinction between teaching, research and action is being erased.

Since it opened eight years ago, the Santa Cruz campus has been involved in environmental issues. Environmental studies were available at UCSC mostly in the form of interdisciplinary courses sponsored by the individual colleges of the Santa Cruz collegiate system.

In the fall of 1971, Kresge College, the sixth residential college in the Santa Cruz System, opened with 300 students and an academic theme of "Man and his Environment."

The program will continue to seek outside funds to develop an environmental center which is a hub of varied activity. Top priority goes to student research projects, student internships, and field opportunities.

As the environmental studies program grows into a full fledged center, it will be more able to meet its primary goal: educating its students and the public in the analysis of environmental problems and in carrying those problems through to solution to the public arena. When Kresge enlarges its facilities, environmental studies hopes that an environmental lawyer, a professional in environmental design, and a demographer will be added to the faculty. With those additions, the program will be able to draw on a very complete environmental faculty housed in a dozen different disciplines.

In addition to the program in environmental studies, the University of California, Santa Cruz is in the planning stages of a series of horticulture courses. The University is also in the process of planning an organic gardening and organic farming course.

For further information, contact:

Richard A. Cooley, Chairman
Committee on Environmental Studies
University of California, Santa Cruz
Santa Cruz, California 95060

CASE WESTERN RESERVE UNIVERSITY
Cleveland, Ohio

URBAN AND ENVIRONMENTAL STUDIES

The city is the central topic of Urban and Environmental Studies. The aim of the program is to examine and understand the city, its functions, its design and its people.

The broad field of urban studies contains many different areas for specialized research. An interdisciplinary curriculum allows students to study a specific subject as it applies to some aspect of the city environment.

A wide range of education opportunities exists in the program due to the participation of other departments and faculty of the University. An advisory committee of both faculty and students participate in the preparation of curriculum and other activities.

Students can structure their program of studies to fit individual educational goals. The program may prepare a student to deal with the urban environment in the professions of architecture, education, engineering, management, medicine and sociology, or in graduate study in the social and behavioral sciences.

Special emphasis is placed on understanding the inter-relationships of many urban conditions.

Students qualify for the B.A. degree in Urban and Environmental Studies by successful completion of fourteen courses. Nine of these are elective, though restricted to social and scientific areas.

Student participation in curriculum and program planning is not only encouraged but solicited.

Metropolitan Cleveland is the laboratory of the program, and field trips are an important part of studies. There, many types of urban phenomena come under detailed observation: retail shopping facilities, wholesale distribution systems, light and heavy industry, education, recreation, neighborhoods, and architecture, government, circulation and transport, housing and housing patterns, and cultural institutions.

Independent or group research is undertaken and reported on during the senior year. Often these seminars take the shape of a group action research project, such as the actual establishment of a neighborhood day-care center for children, assistance in the design of an economic development program, or working to improve the public housing environment.

A limited number of internships with city agencies during Intersession and the Summer Session are available to students in the program. Volunteer work is widely available in the areas of tutoring, recreation, block organization, nonprofit housing projects, civic organization for specific objectives, and area councils.

EARTH ENVIRONMENTAL SCIENCES

The new undergraduate program in Earth Environmental Sciences (EES) will operate through the Department of Geology and in cooperation with the Department of Biology and the Fluid, Thermal and Aerospace Sciences Division in the School of Engineering. Various options associated with this program will allow some specialization in the environmental aspects of geobiology, geochemistry, geophysical fluid mechanics, or geology.

Completion of the program in EES would lead to the award of the degree of Bachelor of Science for Case students. The program includes 25 hours of course work in the earth environmental sciences and 22 hours of basic science.

For further information, contact:

Allen Fonoroff, Chairman
Division of Interdisciplinary Studies in Social
Science
Crawford Hall
Case Western Reserve University
Cleveland, Ohio 44106

CEDAR CREST COLLEGE
(School for Women)
Allentown, Pennsylvania

ENVIRONMENTAL STUDIES

Cedar Crest College has a multidisciplinary major focusing upon the quality of the environment: its biological, political, and social aspects and its moral and aesthetic implications for man. It is designed to give impetus to the search for an environmental ethic and to serve as a catalyst in developing ecological awareness and courses of action. It will enable individuals to become knowledgeable about the environment and man's responsibility to it and at the same time it will train them to fill positions in environmental education, design, research, management and urbanology.

For further information, contact:

Cedar Crest College
Allentown, Pennsylvania 18104

CENTRAL WASHINGTON STATE COLLEGE
Ellensburg, Washington

INTERDEPARTMENTAL MAJOR

CWSC does not offer a major in environmental science. Instead, the college offers the environmentally-minded student an opportunity to pursue his interests through the interdepartmental major program.

This program enables the student to select his area of specialization from the different departments on campus.

For further information, contact:

Central Washington State College
Ellensburg, Washington 98926

CHICO STATE COLLEGE
Chico, California

SCHOOL OF NATURAL SCIENCES

Plans are well advanced for establishment of a Bachelor of Arts degree in Environmental Studies at Chico State College.

At present there is no separate major in Environmental Science although a student can, within a number of departments, specialize in Environmental Science and choose courses from several fields to satisfy degree requirements for his particular major.

For further information, contact:

Chico State College
School of Natural Sciences
Chico, California 95926

UNIVERSITY OF CINCINNATI
Cincinnati, Ohio

CIVIL AND ENVIRONMENTAL ENGINEERING

The University of Cincinnati offers a B.S. curriculum in the combined field of Civil and Environmental Engineering. It is an engineering program and degree.

For further information, contact:

> Louis M. Laushey
> Civil & Environmental Engineering Department
> University of Cincinnati
> Cincinnati, Ohio 45221

CLARKSON COLLEGE OF TECHNOLOGY
Potsdam, New York

DEPARTMENT OF CIVIL ENGINEERING

The curriculum in Civil Engineering at Clarkson College places a strong emphasis on the environmental problems of the future. In order to do this, the program provides the prospective engineer with the fundamental principles of civil engineering. In this manner, the curriculum will enable him to cope with the unknown environmental problems of the future.

ENVIRONMENTAL SCIENCE AND ENGINEERING

A student who wishes to pursue an education in environmental engineering need not be restricted to the Department of Civil Engineering. He may pursue this education by enrolling in any one of Clarkson's engineering departments (chemical, civil, electrical, or mechanical). These departments offer the student a chance to attain knowledge of our environmental problems and give him an opportunity to apply the knowledge that he has acquired to a specific environmental problem.

Students may take one specific environmental problem and convert it into a student project. Some examples of previous student projects are:

> Design of emission control device for Wankel engine.

Design of environmental data transmission systems.

Computer modeling of urban air environments.

Computer optimization of refuse collection systems.

Ammonia stripping from wastewaters.

Water quality in St. Lawrence River.

For further information, contact:

Director of Admissions
Clarkson College of Technology
Potsdam, New York 13676

CLEVELAND STATE UNIVERSITY
Cleveland, Ohio

ENVIRONMENTAL SCIENCES

There are presently more than 120 courses in environmental studies offered in 14 departments at Cleveland State University.

Students may earn Bachelor's degrees in environmental sciences in a number of departments such as Biology, Chemistry and Geology by selecting appropriate elective courses. Students in the Bioengineering program of the Chemical Engineering Department may choose an environmental emphasis.

Students interested in the interactions of the social and natural sciences may major in Urban Studies and emphasize environmental studies through their selection of elective courses.

The Division of Environmental Sciences is cooperating with the Biology Department in offering special training leading to a B.S. in Biology and professional certification as an Environmental Health Specialist (Sanitarian).

The Division of Environmental Sciences is planning a Master's degree program which may be inaugurated in 1972. At present, it offers seven courses which can be applied toward an advanced degree in other departments. In Biology, a student interested in environmental studies may earn an M.S. through one of three programs, (1) straight course work, (2) courses and a research thesis or (3) courses and a project. The project option may be particularly attractive to teachers. They may earn graduate credit for certain approved activities associated with their job such as development of environmental studies curriculum material.

In Chemistry, a student may earn an M.S. in Chemistry with a concentration in Environmental Chemistry. Chemical Engineering offers an Environmental Engineering Option.

In Urban Studies, a graduate student may choose to emphasize environmental studies while earning the M.S.

CONTINUING EDUCATION

The Division of Continuing Education plans to offer a series of seven courses leading to a Professional Certificate in Environmental Management. These courses do not carry academic degree credit.

For further information, contact:

Dr. Robert Rolan, Head
Division of Environmental Sciences
Institute of Urban Studies
Cleveland State University
Cleveland, Ohio

COLBY COLLEGE
Waterville, Maine

ENVIRONMENTAL STUDIES

The program is a multidisciplinary major offered through the Division of Natural Sciences.

The academic aims are intended to provide students with . . .

(1) an understanding of interactions within ecosystems
(2) an appreciation for the contributions which different disciplines make to environmental studies
(3) an awareness about the roles of individuals and institutions that impinge on the environment
(4) a working experience with some aspect of the local or regional environment

For further information, contact:

Biology Department
Colby College
Waterville, Maine 04901

COLLEGE OF THE ATLANTIC
Mount Desert Island, Maine

HUMAN ECOLOGY

College of the Atlantic is a small, coeducational institution awarding the Bachelor of Arts Degree in Human Ecology. Although the aim of the College is to provide a broadly based education for its students, the educational format departs considerably from those of traditional liberal arts colleges. Rather than offering a random assortment of disciplines from which a student may sample, the College is offering a curriculum organized around a central theme, Human Ecology.

The College of the Atlantic was incorporated in July 1969 as a nondenominational, private, coeducational college. It was conceived by the original Trustees, a small group of concerned Mount Desert Island residents from different walks of life, who sought to bring increased intellectual diversity, environmental awareness and economic stability to Mount Desert Island. These trustees leased a twenty-one acre estate on Frenchman's Bay as a site for the College and in January, 1970 appointed a president, Edward G. Kaelber formerly Associate Dean at the Harvard Graduate School of Education. 1970 and 1971 were devoted to intensive planning and fund raising. Early in the planning human ecology, or the interrelationship of man and his environment, was selected as the unifying theme of the curriculum. The original Board of Trustees, realizing that they did not have the range of talents and experience necessary to launch and sustain a college, gave the president a free hand to expand and strengthen the Board which now includes a number of nationally prominent scientists and educators.

During the summer of 1971 a pilot program brought 13 students and three faculty members to the college to test and evaluate certain aspects of the program. Working together with the Administration, a number of Trustees and members of the community (particularly professional staff from the Jackson Laboratory, the Mount Desert Island Biological Laboratory, Acadia National Park and the Maine Coast Heritage Trust), the participants of the summer program began to test the feasibility of developing an undergraduate program based on a concern for a particular environmental problem. The evaluation of the summer experience provided valuable clues about both difficulties and advantages in a problem centered curriculum.

Although the aim of the College is to provide a liberal education it will differ in a number of respects from traditional liberal arts colleges. First, the curriculum being developed is both solid and refreshingly novel. The liberal education at the College of the Atlantic is built around a concern for problems of human ecology or the interrelationship of man and his environment. An examination of environmental problems has been chosen as the core of the curriculum not only because of the urgency of these problems (which makes them "relevant" in the narrower sense), but because their very complexity provides the means for developing those habits of thought and feeling necessary for coping with a changing world.

They anticipate that a somewhat inductive approach, with the feeling that beginning with a specific problem will help students to realize the complexity of environmental/societal problems; that if students are to get beyond superficial understanding of problems, and if they are to make a serious contribution toward solutions, they must focus on a particular aspect; that they must constantly strive to find ways of combining their strengths and perspectives with those of others.

It is their view that actually engaging in some aspect of the workings of society can provide young people with a valuable perspective on themselves, and on the world in which they must play a role. Most of their students will spend a portion of their time (most frequently after their second year of residence) in paid internships or apprenticeships for which credit toward the degree will be given.

The college's ties to the community will go beyond offering special courses for residents. Some citizens of the area will serve as *ad hoc* faculty members working with students and regular faculty members as they explore environmental problems. During the summer 1971 pilot program members of the community (particularly members of the staff of the Jackson Laboratory, the M.D.I. Biological Laboratory, Acadia National Park and the Maine Coast Heritage Trust) joined in discussions of the particular environmental question to which we were directing our attention.

The objective of the College of the Atlantic is to embody its philosophy in a program which will develop the student in three major areas:

(1) Values, attitudes and knowledge necessary to guide the formulation of ideas and decisions which will ensure the enhancement of our quality of life and the survival of all species of life.

(2) The ability to understand the point of view of others and to communicate one's own ideas.

(3) A particular expertise or competency in some area which will enable the student to become effective in a key area relevant to human ecology.

For further information, contact:

College of the Atlantic
Box 3
Bar Harbor, Maine 04609

COLGATE UNIVERSITY
Hamilton, New York

ENVIRONMENTAL SCIENCE

The programs at Colgate dealing either directly or indirectly with Environmental Science are offered through the services of the Biology Department. It is possible at Colgate to develop a concentration with emphasis on environmental problems.

For further information, contact:

Director of Admissions
Colgate University
Hamilton, New York 13346

THE UNIVERSITY OF CONNECTICUT
Storrs, Connecticut

NATURAL RESOURCE CONSERVATION

The College of Agriculture and Natural Resources offers a baccalaureate program in Natural Resource Conservation which serves to meet the interests of many students concerned with maintaining the quality of the environment.

The curriculum contains few required courses and provides students considerable flexibility in developing a program of study specific to their own interests and objectives.

For further information, contact:

John P. H. Brand
Associate Dean
College of Agriculture and Natural Resources
The University of Connecticut
Storrs, Connecticut 06268

CORNELL UNIVERSITY
Ithaca, New York

ENVIRONMENTAL EDUCATION PROGRAM

The aim of this program is to train a student who will be strong in the subject matter of biology, ecology, conservation and who will possess the communication skills necessary for a successful career. Each student will take approximately 50 hours in basic sciences; this background will be supported by courses in education and communication skills such as lecturing, writing, illustrating and exhibit designing. Students are thereby prepared for professional careers in environmental interpretation and nature center work, museum educational programs, outdoor education, state and private conservation organizations, Audubon societies, professional scouting and publications dealing with natural history, conservation, and environmental education.

NATURAL RESOURCES PROGRAM

Students may elect one of five programs within the Natural Resources Program. The three science programs give preparation for graduate work, but they may be modified for students who wish to terminate their study at the bachelor's level and go directly into a professional management career. The curriculum in Outdoor Recreation is intended for managers or planners of land and water devoted primarily to recreational use. The program in environmental conservation is a general educational program designed to prepare citizens to understand their bio-physical environment and man's impact on it. It blends the biological, physical, social sciences and humanities so that a sound base is provided for the pursuit of graduate studies in many areas having to do with man's management of his environment.

In addition to these programs, Cornell University also publishes two ecologically oriented newsletters. Both *Conservation Comments* and *Ecology News* discuss current environment-preserving activities within the Cornell University campus.

For further information, contact:

> Dr. Richard B. Fischer
> 16 Stone Hall
> Cornell University
> Ithaca, New York 14850

ECOLOGY HOUSE

The Ecology House was founded on the principle that man is an integral and equal part of the world environment; that he can function as a member of a natural ecosystem, rather than as its would-be conqueror; and that through a fuller understanding of ecological processes and their practical applications, he can immensely improve the quality of life on earth. The first and foremost objective of the House, therefore, is to prove that people can function as members of a natural ecosystem without sacrificing all of the benefits of modern technology.

In accomplishing this objective, the Ecology House hopes to (1) provide an example of an environmentally-conscious existence, with group interaction and cooperation provided for within a common living unit; (2) endeavor to prepare the public, special interest groups and individuals for an ecologically sound way of life; (3) interpret the ecological consequences of man's activities from philosophical, technical and applied points of view; (4) utilize the tremendous diversity of Cornell University, with graduate, undergraduate and faculty residents from many different disciplines, and to act as a liaison between the environmental and technological sciences; (5) act as a meeting place, project coordination headquarters and information pool for other similar organizations, and promote the founding of similar living units at other universities and provide them with the knowledge gained through experience; and (6) create an intimate awareness of the relationship between the quality of the environment and the quality of human life, and above all, ensure the survival of the human species by ensuring the survival of the ecological systems on which man depends.

The Ecology House is also actively involved in the recycling of glass, newspaper, aluminum and white paper. For further information, contact:

Ecology House
Residential Club
Cornell University
Ithaca, New York 14850

DANA COLLEGE
Blair, Nebraska

ENVIRONMENTAL STUDIES

Recognizing that environmental problems arise from a complex of advancing technologies and increasing human populations, and that these arise from scientific, economic, and social factors in our society, the program at Dana College is deliberately composed of courses representing a number of academic areas. A seminar, meeting each week throughout the school year, attempts to integrate the separate disciplines to show the inter-relations of science, economics, and social considerations. The major includes eleven courses and a related supporting area (selected by the student to meet his individual vocational interest) is recommended.

For further information, contact:

George E. Grube
Dana College
Blair, Nebraska 68008

DARTMOUTH COLLEGE
Hanover, New Hampshire

ENVIRONMENTAL STUDIES PROGRAM

The principal mission of the Dartmouth Environmental Studies Program is to provide an opportunity for undergraduates to assess the seriousness and complexities of environmental problems. Two secondary objectives of the program are to aid in public education programs on environmental issues, and to stimulate interdisciplinary research on environmental problems at the college.

The program currently does not represent an area of specialization, or a "major", but is organized to serve as a kind of "minor"to be associated with any other major in the college. This is implemented through a curricular arrangement termed a "modified major" which combines four courses from one area (environmental studies) with six courses from another area. It is the current philosophy of program members that this arrangement permits students to develop competence in a traditionally recognized discipline which can be brought to bear on analysis and rectification of environmental situations.

One of the original goals of the Environmental Studies Program was to stimulate the traditional academic departments to formulate and offer their own environmentally oriented courses. Many departments have begun such courses or implemented their old courses with new subject matter. Anthropology, Art, Biology, Chemistry, Earth Sciences, Economics, Engineering, Geography, Government, Psychology and Sociology have all instituted environmental courses.

The program is also associated with certain extracurricular activities and some research on campus. The Dartmouth Outing Club, the largest organized activity on campus, has recently added an Environmental Studies Division, which is the student activist environmental group on campus. The Division has promoted a recycling campaign, done research on various regional and campus environmental problems, and has organized an Environmental Studies Library. The library has books on all environmental topics and contains a complete collection of journals, newsletters, magazines, government documents and regional newspaper files for the past two years. The Environmental Studies Program makes use of the library's resources, maintains reserve readings there, and cooperates with the activities of the DOC Environmental Studies Division, often cosponsoring programs and lectures on campus. Student research in Environmental Studies has been made possible by a grant from the Richard King Mellon Foundation to be used to organize and conduct practical work in the field of conservation and environmental science.

For further information, contact:

Darthmouth College
Environmental Studies Program
52 Robinson Hall
Hanover, New Hampshire 03755

DePAUL UNIVERSITY
Chicago, Illinois

ENVIRONMENTAL ANALYSIS

De Paul University currently offers an Environmental Analysis Program through its Chemistry Department. The program leads to a B.S. degree in Chemistry.

For further information, contact:

De Paul University
College of Liberal Arts and Sciences
2323 North Seminary Avenue
Chicago, Illinois 60614

DOANE COLLEGE
Crete, Nebraska

ENVIRONMENTAL STUDY MAJOR

The environmental study major at Doane College is structured so that every student enrolled in the program completes a liberal arts background and a core of courses in the sciences and social sciences to provide a broad base for further environmental science. During the last two years the student develops an emphasis in biology, chemistry or the social sciences, depending on his personal interest in various aspects of the environmental crisis.

For further information, contact:

Doane College
Crete, Nebraska 68333

DREXEL UNIVERSITY
Philadelphia, Pennsylvania

ENVIRONMENTAL ENGINEERING

At the present time, Drexel University does not have any major at the baccalaureate level in Environmental Science. However, there are several established programs which include opportunities to take elective courses related to the environment.

One of the required courses in this curriculum is Environmental Engineering. This basic course can then be followed by up to six elective courses chosen from Sanitary Engineering, Water Resources & Supply, Hydrology, as well as courses from the Environmental Engineering & Science Graduate Program. Other Engineering curricula have this elective feature also. Many faculty from Drexel teach in the Environmental Engineering & Science multidisciplinary graduate program.

For further information, contact:

Richard E. Woodring
Associate Dean of Engineering
Drexel University
Philadelphia, Pennsylvania 19104

EAST TENNESSEE STATE UNIVERSITY
Johnson City, Tennessee

ENVIRONMENTAL HEALTH

The Department of Environmental Health has three basic programs. The programs are: an Annual Public Health Sanitation School, a baccalaureate degree leading to the degree, Bachelor of Science in Environmental Health (B.S.E.H.), and a graduate program leading to the professional degree, Master of Science in Environmental Health (M.S.E.H.)

For further information, contact:

Professor Phillip M. Cooper
Department of Environmental Health
College of Health
East Tennessee State University
Johnson City, Tennessee 37601

GEORGIA INSTITUTE OF TECHNOLOGY
Atlanta, Georgia

ENVIRONMENTAL RESOURCES CENTER

Through its activities, the Environmental Resources Center fosters coordinated programs of education and research related to environmental management. It places special emphasis on multidisciplinary, problem-focused programs which involve interaction between science and technology, socio-economic systems, and the natural environment.

The ERC does not offer a designated degree. Instead, it encourages the development of multidepartmental curricula augmented by special courses and directed studies in the interdisciplinary aspects of environmental problems. It stimulates and coordinates Georgia Tech's involvement in off-campus and service activities related to environmental resources. It seeks funds to support education and research in relevant subject areas, and it provides leadership and coordination for interdisciplinary teams, committees, short courses and conferences, and publications. As one of its most important functions, the Environmental Resources Center serves as a center for the storage and exchange of information regarding ongoing research and educational programs and public service activities.

For further information, contact:

Carl E. Kindsvater, Assistant Director
Environmental Resources Center
Georgia Institute of Technology
Atlanta, Georgia 30332

GUSTAVUS ADOLPHUS COLLEGE
Saint Peter, Minnesota

ENVIRONMENTAL STUDIES

An environmental studies distributive major is offered at Gustavus Adolphus College. That major includes 12 courses including certain biology and environmental studies courses, which are required. A student must also have some work in the departments of chemistry, economics, geography, geology and sociology.

For further information, contact:

> Owen E. Sammelson
> Director of Admissions
> Gustavus Adolphus College
> Saint Peter, Minnesota 56082

HAMPSHIRE COLLEGE
Amherst, Massachusetts
EXPERIMENTAL ENVIRONMENTAL STUDIES

At Hampshire College, a new and frankly experimental school in Amherst, Massachusetts, there's little time for sitting back and bawling out displeasure with the corrupted environment. Everyone's too busy building an environmentally sane, if not safe, community.

Broadly, the school states as one of its major goals: "To develop a campus where educational, esthetic, and ecological designs support and enhance one another." The point is, nobody knows how exactly to do this, so the school, the faculty and the students are working it out together. Hampshire shares the Connecticut River Valley of central Massachusetts with four prestige schools, Amherst, Smith, Mt. Holyoke and the University of Massachusetts, and shares some of these schools' faculties and facilities. Hampshire is a well-funded school constantly searching for ways to keep costs down, but quality high. That "natural-is-best" follows isn't surprising.

As the college grows its farmland will be put to a variety of new uses, each with its special impact on the ecology of the area.

Hampshire wants its students to learn and use proper survey techniques for a comprehensive inventory of the present 550-acre campus, so they'll know the quantities and qualities of the ecosystem they're dealing with.

There are a number of working farms still located on Hampshire's land. The students want the farmers to stop using chemical fertilizers and pesticides, but the farmers are a little leery of what might happen without pesticides. The school may try to encourage the farmers to build up their land organically before stopping pesticide use, or it may devise another course—but throughout, the school emphasized the human approach that took into full account these farmers' need to make a livelihood and their right to be apprehensive.

Other groups are now studying the school's building design and location in relation to the surrounding woods, open space, and other buildings. Most of the four and five story living and classroom buildings now open or going up are shaped to echo the lines of a nearby dominant mountain. Though the buildings are high, their contour reinforces the natural design.

There are plans for experimental creation of forest borders, hedgerows, and other wildlife habitats to encourage the wildlife to live as close to the college center as possible.

These attempts already show in the appearance of Hampshire. Coming from the highway up the long driveway, there's nothing but trees and fields in sight for a quarter mile.

A group is studying alternatives to salt and plowing for snow control, and to asphalt and concrete roads and walks. The idea isn't to conquer nature but to live with her.

Students are looking into composting procedures for the school's solid organic waste and the recycling or disposal of nondegradables. They contacted the Amherst sewage treatment plant but found the sludge had been treated with ferric chloride to make it settle. They decided to test it experimentally first, to determine the effects of ferric chloride, before using it on the land.

Another group is designing a microbiological sewage treatment facility for the college. It hopes eventually to reclaim the school's sludge.

In other words, Hampshire College is aiming to become as closed an ecosystem as possible within the framework of its function.

ENVIRONMENTAL QUALITY PROGRAM

This program consists of lectures, seminars, and research projects concerning the problems of environmental deterioration.

Students enter this department with an awareness of the rapidly deteriorating environment, the neglect of air and water quality and misuse of soils and other natural resources.

For further information, contact:

> Hampshire College
> Amherst, Massachusetts 01002

HARTWICK COLLEGE
Oneonta, New York
INDIVIDUAL STUDENT PROGRAMS

Hartwick College does not currently offer a multi-disciplinary environmental science major. However, it is possible for a student to obtain a baccalaureate degree by successfully completing a program of study which he has developed with the approval of the Committee on Individual Student Programs. The committee helps the student determine if the college possesses the faculty and material resources required for the proposed program. In at least two instances, student-developed programs emphasizing the area of human ecology have been approved. These obviously are multi-disciplinary in scope and draw upon the faculties from the physical and life sciences, social and behavioral sciences, and the humanities.

For further information, contact:

> Director of Admissions
> Hartwick College
> Oneonta, New York 13820

UNIVERSITY OF HAWAII
Honolulu, Hawaii
SURVIVAL-PLUS PROGRAM

Survival-Plus is an innovative program at the University of Hawaii which allows a student to organize all of his undergraduate training around the major crises that threaten extinction to the human race. It is ecological in the sense that it examines the complex interactions of man and thus students will examine the problems of human alienation, war, social and economic inequity, etc., as well as those of pollution, overpopulation, urban decay, and the depletion of natural resources. In short, the program addresses itself to the central question: "How can the human race survive under conditions which might make survival worthwhile?"

For further information, contact:

> Coordinator, Survival Plus Program
> Dean Hall
> University of Hawaii
> 2450 Campus Road
> Honolulu, Hawaii 96822

HEIDELBERG COLLEGE
Tiffin, Ohio

ENVIRONMENTAL SCIENCE EMPHASIS

Heidelberg College has an environmental science emphasis within its regular course offerings. Students are encouraged to develop from the departments of biology, physics, economics, and other departments a series of courses which will permit them to emphasize environmental science. A biology major, for example, would have an environmental emphasis and his cognate courses in areas such as physics and chemistry would support both biology and the environmental emphasis.

For some time Heidelberg has had a Sandusky River project. This is an undergraduate research project which has been funded through college funds, National Science Foundation grants, and private foundation money. The emphasis on the project is to study, over a period of years, a small river in northwestern Ohio which defines a drainage basin with a population of about 250,000. Many of the students who have been interested in environmental science have been involved during the school year and in the summer working on this project. Heidelberg College was one of the first colleges in the United States to receive National Science Foundation support for student-originated research in environmental science.

For further information, write:

> Arthur R. Porter, Jr.
> Dean of the College
> Heidelberg College
> Tiffin, Ohio 44883

HILLSDALE COLLEGE
Hillsdale, Michigan

ENVIRONMENTAL STUDIES

Hillsdale College offers an interdisciplinary field of concentration in Environmental Studies.

For further information, contact:

> Hillsdale College
> Hillsdale, Michigan 49242

HIRAM COLLEGE
Hiram, Ohio

ENVIRONMENTAL STUDIES

Through both established areas of concentration planned by individual departments, and individually designed areas of concentration planned by the student and his advisor, the student at Hiram College is given a chance to both explore and develop his environmental interests. The student is encouraged to plan his education directly in the sciences and, through his area of concentration, enroll in those courses which would supplement his environmental interest. As a student learns environmental science at Hiram College, he learns it in many ways. The student learns not only by what he studies, but also how he integrates the entire learning opportunity into an environmental consideration.

For further information, contact:

> Hiram College
> Hiram, Ohio 44234

HOPE COLLEGE
Holland, Michigan

INSTITUTE FOR ENVIRONMENTAL QUALITY

Hope College has within its campus an Institute for Environmental Quality. The primary purpose of this Institute is to coordinate multidisciplinary research on matters involving environmental quality especially on water problems.

For further information, contact:

> Hope College
> Holland, Michigan 49423

HUXLEY COLLEGE OF ENVIRONMENTAL STUDIES
A Division of Western Washington State College
Bellingham, Washington

MULTIDISCIPLINARY STUDY

Understanding man's ecological relations demands study among established disciplines. Huxley College, consequently, offers multidisciplinary study encompassing all of the physical, biological and social dimensions of environmental problems. The contemporary demand for educational relevance requires that Huxley graduates understand not only the workings of our environment but also ways in which environmental order may be maintained. Problem-oriented study is stressed at Huxley, and concepts from the classroom are applied to specific situations.

Huxley's curriculum is based upon a common core program, problem series and seminars in environmental studies.

CORE COURSES

These courses are designed to give all students a common background in environmental concepts essential for comprehension of man; his natural, physical and social environment; and his reliance and influence on these environments. The core courses are action-oriented, combining laboratory and field experiments, lectures, readings and discussions. Introductory courses in biology, chemistry and physics are recommended as prerequisites to these core courses.

PROBLEM SERIES

Students at Huxley College are expected to carry out independent study pertaining to environmental issues. The problem series is undertaken with advice and assistance from one or more tutors from the Huxley faculty. It may be several individual problem investigations or a series of steps in a major investigation; it may take the form of a library, laboratory, or community experience. This investigation, observation and interpretation must be followed by the student's recorded statement (written, taped, filmed, or graphically portrayed) demonstrating his process of situation analysis and interpretation, his prognosis and his proposed steps to action.

SEMINARS

Seminars offer a meeting ground for a free exchange of information and discussion between faculty and students. They allow for detailed studies of particular topics and are a testing ground for new areas of potential campus concern. They serve to increase interaction between students and faculty of different concentrations. They allow the Huxley community a further opportunity to gain knowledge in aspects of concentrations and environmental issues other than their own studies. Students normally participate in one seminar per quarter.

CONCENTRATIONS

In addition to the common program, students work in recognized areas of environmental concern called concentrations. These concentrations focus on general environmental problems which draw upon a number of specialized disciplines for solutions. In addition to working in a concentration (selected not later than one quarter after entering Huxley and preferably at time of entry), students are expected to develop competence in a classical discipline, such as sociology or chemistry.

Huxley students may develop individual concentrations to suit particular needs and interests; such programs are approved through an "academic contract." Most students find that the concentrations offered afford considerable flexibility in their academic programs. At present the following concentrations are offered:

> Ecosystems Analysis
> Environmental Control
> Environmental Planning
> Environmental Health
> Marine Resources
> Environmental Education
> Human Ecology

For further information, contact:

> Huxley College
> A Division of
> Western Washington State College
> Bellingham, Washington 98225

IDAHO STATE UNIVERSITY
Pocatello, Idaho

ENVIRONMENTAL PHYSICS
Idaho State has a major in Environmental Physics.

For further information, contact:

Mike Standley
Assistant Registrar
Idaho State University
Pocatello, Idaho 83201

UNIVERSITY OF IDAHO
Moscow, Idaho

COLLEGE OF FORESTRY, WILDLIFE, AND RANGE SCIENCES
The academic objective of the College of Forestry, Wildlife and Range Sciences is to acquire competence for entry into professional careers in resource science and management. Each of the curricula offered by the College, therefore, assures the student an acquaintance with the physical, biological, and social sciences and the humanities. This provides the student with the preparation he needs for his scientific-professional courses dealing with the use of forest and range lands and related resources.

WATER RESOURCES RESEARCH INSTITUTE
This institute, established in 1963, has the following objectives:

(1) To increase, improve and coordinate the efforts of the various university divisions and departments concerned with water resources research by assisting in (a) defining problem areas; (b) encouraging and promoting team efforts between different disciplines; and (c) assisting in the planning and implementation of interdisciplinary research in cooperation with federal, state and private agencies.

(2) To strengthen and coordinate undergraduate and graduate programs and course offerings so that the university can supply well-trained teachers and

leaders capable of coping with the complex water problems at the local, state, regional and national levels by (a) encouraging the use of improved teaching techniques and the upgrading of the staff; (b) developing logical sequences of courses to maximize teaching efforts; (c) conducting interdisciplinary seminars to acquaint students and faculty with the broad aspects of water resources; and (d) bringing outstanding authorities to the campus for seminars and conferences.

(3) To gather, disseminate and coordinate ideas and research findings between the university and various federal and state agencies and local and civic groups interested in water resources by (a) publishing quality reports of findings; (b) sponsoring or appearing at meetings and workshops to serve all interests; and (c) building and maintaining a library which will be a central source of information to all concerned.

For further information, contact:

C. C. Warnick, Director
34 Engineering Building
University of Idaho
Moscow, Idaho 83843

ILLINOIS INSTITUTE OF TECHNOLOGY
Chicago, Illinois

ENVIRONMENTAL ENGINEERING

The Department of Environmental Engineering at Illinois Institute of Technology does not currently offer an undergraduate program in Environmental Science. Civil Engineering students, however, have available an option in Environmental Engineering, which involves three courses in the Department of Environmental Engineering and one biology course.

For further information, contact:

Dr. Roger A. Minear
Assistant Professor
Environmental Engineering
Illinois Institute of Technology
Chicago, Illinois 60616

UNIVERSITY OF ILLINOIS AT URBANA-CHAMPAIGN
Urbana, Illinois

INDEPENDENT STUDY

At the present time the University of Illinois does not have a formal undergraduate major in environmental science. However, many students are tailoring individual programs dealing with environmental concerns under the auspices of the New Independent Plans of Study Program.

Through this program a student will be able to specialize in environmental science by selecting courses on this subject from the numerous courses the university offers.

For further information, contact:

> College of Liberal Arts and Sciences
> Office of the Dean
> 294 Lincoln Hall
> Urbana, Illinois 61801

INDIANA UNIVERSITY
Bloomington, Indiana

ENVIRONMENTAL STUDIES

Environmental Studies at Indiana University is an interdepartmental program designed to introduce students to environmental problems associated with modern civilizations. The program includes a multidisciplinary study of the effects of population growth, resources utilization, energy generation, and agricultural systems as well as of the emergence of environment as a focus for public policy.

Students who major in this program must also complete a major in an established discipline as well as in Environmental Studies. Two options are available for the Environmental Studies major. Option I is presented primarily for students in biological and physical sciences, whereas Option II is proposed primarily for students in social or behavioral sciences or humanities.

For the benefit of high school students, it is here noted that two years of high school algebra and one year of geometry, or their equivalent are assumed as background in this program and most related departmental programs. For further information, contact:

Craig Nelson
Department of Zoology
Indiana University
Bloomington, Indiana 47401

INTERNATIONAL ECOSYSTEMS UNIVERSITY
Berkeley, California

INTERDISCIPLINARY ENVIRONMENTAL STUDY

International Ecosystems University (IEU) is an independent, non-sectarian institution of higher learning dedicated to the following purposes:

(1) To provide comprehensive transdisciplinary programs of professional study at the undergraduate, graduate and professional levels for persons preparing themselves for careers in the environmental and ecosystems sciences.

(2) To provide continuing education for persons in all walks of life engaged in learning for their own personal growth, enabling them to continue developing flexible and innovative solutions to the ever-changing and increasing problems in the maintenance of a complex life-supporting environment.

(3) To enrich the interpersonal as well as educational experiences of its students and to contribute to the growth of the world community by creating an environment for education, research and action to deal with the environmental and socio-cultural problems now affecting our world on a local, regional, national and supra-national basis.

(4) To develop in its students awareness and a sense of personal, social, civic responsibility, as well as leadership qualities essential for the creative evolution of our society.

(5) To establish the IEU through recruiting and offering equal educational opportunities for qualified

persons regardless of race, sex, religion, or national origin.

For further information, contact:

Robert R. Wiseman, Administrative Officer
Forum International
2905 Benvenue
Berkeley, California 94705

THE JOHNS HOPKINS UNIVERSITY
Baltimore, Maryland

ENVIRONMENTAL ENGINEERING

Johns Hopkins University has a program in Environmental Engineering.

For further information, contact:

The Johns Hopkins University
Department of Environmental Engineering
Baltimore, Maryland 21218

JOHNSON STATE COLLEGE
Johnson, Vermont

ENVIRONMENTAL CURRICULUM

Johnson State College has a concentration in Environmental Science, which, when teamed with a traditional area of study, will constitute an academic major. Specifically they will turn out students trained in any of their present fields who have additionally studied the environment. For instance, a person can, under this proposal, achieve a major consisting of a minor in environmental studies coupled with a minor from any other field. An important second option also available to students would involve those in elementary education. They could choose environmental studies as the concentration area they are now required to have under new elementary education curriculum.

For further information, contact:

Johnson Sate College
Johnson, Vermont 05656

THE UNIVERSITY OF KANSAS
Lawrence, Kansas

ENVIRONMENTAL SYSTEMS AND DESIGN

The University of Kansas has two degree programs concerned with the environment:

a B.S. degree in Systematics and Ecology, and

a B.E.D. degree in Environmental Design.

For further information, contact:

> Admissions Office
> University of Kansas
> Lawrence, Kansas 66044

KANSAS WESLEYAN
Salina, Kansas

SURVIVAL STUDIES PROGRAM

The Survival Studies Program offers a major somewhat different from those offered in most of the college's departments. In fact, no two major programs are exactly alike; the precise content of a major will depend upon the interests and background of the student. Within this context of flexibility the following statements are pertinent.

(1) The student and his advisor will establish a committee to include the student's advisor and two other members of the Survival Studies faculty.

(2) The student and his advisor will then present to the full committee a proposed course of study for the approval of the committee. The committee will also annually review the progress of the student.

(3) The student's program will include the following features:

    (a) The student must meet the college's general education requirements for graduation.

    (b) The student's program must include an acceptable project which will occupy a major portion of the student's time during his junior and senior years at Kansas Wesleyan; the evidence of this effort, normally in the form of a written report, must be presented to and accepted by the Survival Studies faculty during the final semester of the student's residence.

(c) The student will select additional courses particularly relevant to his project.

For further information, contact:

Director of Survival Studies
Kansas Wesleyan
Salina, Kansas 67401

KEARNEY STATE COLLEGE
Kearney, Nebraska

ENVIRONMENTAL STUDIES

Kearney State College has instituted a program of environmental studies. Some of the main objectives are:

(1) To provide courses in environmental studies which assist the students in their understanding of the problems which confront our environment and their effects on society.

(2) To provide a program of study for the student who desires a career in the area of environmental science.

(3) To try to develop an awareness among our students as to their personal responsibility to the environment, with courses that explore the economic, historical, political, psychological, and sociological aspects of the relationship of man to environmental problems.

(4) To promote among students, faculty and personnel interested in and engaged in environmental work, the systematic and scientific study of environmental problems.

For further information, contact:

Dr. Harold Nagel
Kearney State College
Kearney, Nebraska 68847

KIRKLAND HALL JUNIOR COLLEGE
Easton, Maryland

INTERDISCIPLINARY ENVIRONMENTAL STUDY

Kirkland Hall students will have environmental training intermeshed with their regular studies; two-year degrees in ecology and conservation will be granted; and an environmental research center operates as a campus facility.

The work of the research center will eventually help to give advice on specific ecological problems.

The school was established in 1967 on 80 acres of a 700-acre estate bordering the Miles River near the Chesapeake Bay. Barns, homes and milk sheds were turned into campus buildings in the center of a "nature wonderland."

For further information, contact:

> Kirkland Hall Junior College
> Easton, Maryland 21601

LAWRENCE UNIVERSITY
Appleton, Wisconsin

INTERDISCIPLINARY STUDY

Lawrence University has no formal major in Environmental Science. However, students interested in this area can, through their regular interdisciplinary major in the sciences or through a student-designed major, build a program that meets their individual needs. In addition to strong disciplinary programs in biology, geology, chemistry, physics, economics and political science, which might be of interest to students of environmental science, Lawrence University offers many courses in the environmental sciences.

They also have an Environmental Action Committee that is seeking to promote recycling of wastes at the university and to seek university action to minimize deleterious effects of university activities on the environment.

For further information, contact:

> Robert M. Rosenberg
> Professor of Chemistry
> Lawrence University
> Box 1847
> Appleton, Wisconsin 54911

LEHIGH UNIVERSITY
Bethlehem, Pennsylvania

ENVIRONMENTAL SCIENCES

The Environmental Sciences and Resource Management programs at Lehigh University are interdepartmental majors, tailored to fit the individual student's interests. A core of courses is required by all participants. In addition, the other requirements of the University must be satisfied. The total course load totals considerably more than the minimum or average for graduation from Lehigh. This facet tends to eliminate students whose interests are not real, and should result in a sound reputation for the graduates of the program.

For further information, contact:

E. E. MacNamara
Lehigh University
Bethlehem, Pennsylvania 18015

CENTER FOR MARINE AND ENVIRONMENTAL STUDIES

The Center for Marine and Environmental Studies is an interdepartmental research organization with the primary purpose of providing research opportunities in marine science, ocean engineering and environmental studies for faculty and graduate students from several academic departments. The Center also contributes to the undergraduate and graduate teaching programs of the University.

The center is not an academic department, and thus does not offer courses nor award degrees. The staff of the center hold academic appointments and teach in established departments. Graduate students associated with the center are enrolled in and receive their degrees from one of the academic departments—biology, chemistry, geological sciences, physics, or one of the several engineering fields.

Research is emphasized at all levels of graduate study. There are many opportunities for beginning graduate students to cooperate with staff on laboratory and field studies. Advanced students are encouraged to undertake independent and interdisciplinary research problems.

Much of marine science and ocean engineering is learned by actually doing research in the marine environment. Although Lehigh is an inland university, the staff and students of CMES have a wide variety of opportunities to work at sea through arrangements with other institutions. Cooperative programs are active with Woods Hole Oceanographic Institution, the Atlantic Oceanographic Laboratories of NOAA (Miami), Texas A & M University, Duke University, Scripps Institution of Oceanography, Lockheed Ocean Laboratory, and the U.S. Coast Guard. Research projects are active in the Atlantic and Pacific Oceans, the Gulf of Mexico, and Delaware Bay.

Active research projects in environmental studies provide practical experience for graduate students.

For further information, write:

> James M. Parks, Director
> Center for Marine and Environmental Studies
> Lehigh University
> Bethlehem, Pennsylvania 18015

SOUTH JERSEY WETLANDS INSTITUTE
Stone Harbor, New Jersey

The aims of the research and educational programs to be conducted at the South Jersey Wetlands Institute are:

(1) To increase the understanding of the natural processes controlling the wetlands ecosystems through fundamental research;

(2) To investigate the renewability of the natural resources and increase the biotic potential of the area;

(3) To ascertain the effects of disturbances caused by man's activities, and to find methods of minimizing these effects through practical and applied research;

(4) To provide factual scientific information which can serve others as a basis on which to make intelligent decisions for the long range beneficial multiple use of coastal areas;

(5) To train scientists and engineers in methods of solving and of preventing problems in coastal zones;

(6) To educate the general public, both resident and vacationing, as to the importance of wetlands to the general ecology of coastal areas, the need for preserving and enhancing the wetlands in maintaining the aspects of the

coastal zones that make it attractive to residents and vacationers, and what each can do to protect the environment.

For further information, contact:

Dr. Sidney S. Herman, Director
South Jersey Wetlands Institute
Lehigh University
Bethlehem, Pennsylvania 18015

LOUISIANA STATE UNIVERSITY
Baton Rouge, Louisiana

ENVIRONMENTAL DESIGN

The School of Environmental Design at Louisiana State University was established in 1966 bringing together the facilities of Architecture, Landscape Architecture, Construction Technology, Fine Arts and Interior Design. They are hoping to add a program in Regional and Urban Planning in the not too distant future. In uniting these academic units they are placing great emphasis on ecological and environmental impacts of physical development.

In addition to this, the university has programs in Environmental Engineering, Engineering Science, and Environmental Law. They also have outstanding programs in coastal and wetlands studies.

They plan to bring all the departments together, and establish an Environmental Sciences Institute.

For further information, contact:

Gerald J. McLindon, Dean
School of Environmental Design
Louisiana State University
Baton Rouge, Louisiana 70803

UNIVERSITY OF LOUISVILLE
Louisville, Kentucky

HORNER BUD AND WILDLIFE SANCTUARY

This 200-acre tract, a gift to the university, is located upon a plateau about 25 miles from the campus. It is largely covered by second-growth deciduous forest, and it contains streams, steep hillsides, and rolling upland. It serves not only as a wildlife sanctuary, but also as a field laboratory for class trips and for research in plant and animal ecology and natural history.

ENVIRONMENTAL ENGINEERING

The Speed Scientific School, the School of Engineering and Applied Science of the University of Louisville, stands for some definite ideas in education. It is a college that emphasizes engineering as a means of understanding and controlling the forces at work in the world today. This is the dominant idea influencing the point of view of the college.

The University of Louisville offers an interdisciplinary program in Environmental Engineering, designed to train engineers to assist in the total management of a community's environment as it relates especially to its health resources. Emphasis is placed on practical environmental problems and training.

For further information, contact:

University of Louisville,
2301 South Third Street
Louisville, Kentucky 40208

UNIVERSITY OF MAINE AT ORONO
Orono, Maine

DEPARTMENT OF PLANT AND SOIL SCIENCES

The Department of Plant and Soil Sciences at the University of Maine at Orono, participates with several other departments in a Natural Resource curriculum. The options that are available in this program, and that ultimately lead to a B.S. degree in Natural Resource Management are:

(1) *Conservation Technology Engineering*—principles and technology related to conservation of natural resources;

(2) *Resource Economics*—economic and business aspects of resource development;

(3) *Forest Resources*—multiple use and management

of forest lands and conservation of wildlife and habitat;

(4) *Soil and Water Conservation*—(Plant & Soil Science option) soil conservation and hydrology;

(5) *Recreation and Park Management*—management of recreation resources.

The program attempts to meet an increasing need for people in the field of natural resource management to be involved in planning and decision making related to wise use of limited land and water resources. A rapidly increasing population and more leisure time means keener competition by industrial, recreational, and agricultural interests for available land and water.

The Department also has two other environment-related areas in which students may major; Plant Science, and Soil Science. Students in either of these curriculums are provided with a knowledge of basic sciences, soils, plants, landscaping, and ornamental horticulture. The degree awarded is a B.S. in Plant and Soil Sciences. The training received will qualify the students for careers in teaching, extension work, production, and service functions for industry, Soil Conservation Service, and other related government agencies, farming, landscaping, consulting, inspection, communications and sales.

For further information, contact:

University of Maine
Deering Hall
Orono, Maine 04473

MARQUETTE UNIVERSITY
Milwaukee, Wisconsin

ENVIRONMENTAL ENGINEERING

At Marquette University, College of Engineering, there is a program entitled "Environmental Engineering Interdisciplinary Curriculum," administered by the Civil Engineering Department. The core of the program is still a civil engineering curriculum, but in place of many non-environmentally related civil engineering courses, the student is permitted to take courses in biology, chemistry, statistics, economics, anthropology, etc. Upon completion of the program the student receives a Bachelor of Science degree in Civil Engineering, but with a major in environmental engineering. Students who elect to go into the program must begin during the freshman year and take the newly developed course entitled "Introduction to Environmental Engineering."

For more information, contact:

College of Engineering
Department of Civil Engineering
Marquette University
1515 West Wisconsin Avenue
Milwaukee, Wisconsin 53233

MASSACHUSETTS INSTITUTE OF TECHNOLOGY
Cambridge, Massachusetts
ENVIRONMENTAL STUDIES

Environmental studies for undergraduates at MIT are available through a variety of departmental and interdepartmental courses and laboratories which are growing in number. Although there is no separate degree program at either the graduate or undergraduate level, many departments offer educational and research opportunities in those aspects of the environment which are closely related to their own disciplinary interests. Undergraduate students who are uncommitted to any of the standard disciplines may arrange a coordinated program of interdisciplinary environmental study by entering one of the unspecified degree programs sponsored by many of the departments. Undergraduate students who have a disciplinary commitment but wish a coherent minor program of environmental study may do so through use of the unrestricted electives available to them. Departments have appointed advisors on interdisciplinary environmental concentration. Further information, lists of departmental advisors and sample programs of studies on environmental issues are available through the Office of the Provost, Room 3-240.

The Institute has formed an Interdisciplinary Environmental Council whose purpose is to take an overview of all educational and research activities that relate to environmental concerns. The establishment of the Council reflects the recognition that successful education and research in this area required the involvement of a number of disciplines drawing on expertise of many departments. The Council will be available to any group at the Institute for advice and assistance concerning research and educational programs dealing with problems of the environment.

The Council will have continuing responsibility for the formulation of policy on issues that relate to interdisciplinary environmental teaching and research at the Institute. A primary concern of the Council will be to review the development of interdisciplinary educational opportunities both at the undergraduate and graduate level. When appropriate, the Council will take the initiative for the establishment of new educational programs, subjects, seminars, or interdisciplinary research projects. The Council will work closely with the newly created MIT Environmental Laboratory.

For further information, contact:

Massachusetts Institute of Technology
Cambridge, Massachusetts 02139

UNIVERSITY OF MASSACHUSETTS
Amherst, Massachusetts

The University of Massachusetts offers two programs leading to a Bachelor of Science in Environmental Science, backed up by six other environmentally concerned organizations. The two programs:

ENVIRONMENTAL TECHNOLOGY

The Department of Environmental Sciences, as sponsor of this program, maintains that the first step of any environmental research is a biological-chemical inventory, obtainable by using standard scientific method. Therefore, considerable emphasis is placed on methodology. The department offers an apprenticeship program in which the student spends time working in a Water Quality Office Regional Laboratory, rotating through various services to provide practical skills.

A two-year program in Environmental Technology also is offered, leading to a variety of practical skills and an associate degree in Environmental Technology.

For further information, contact:

> Department of Environmental Sciences
> University of Massachusetts
> Amherst, Massachusetts 01002

PLANT AND SOIL SCIENCES

The Department of Plant and Soil Sciences is centered around the concepts of soil management and proper methods of crop planting. Courses include plant nutrition, soil management and fertility, plant culture, crop and variety selection, and harvesting and storage.

Also included, under the Department of Nutrition and Food, is a study of several types of diets, including the "average" American diet, natural-organic foods, and highly processed foods.

For further information, contact:

> Dr. F. W. Southwick
> Department of Plant and Soil Sciences
> University of Massachusetts
> Amherst, Massachusetts 01002

> Peter L. Pellett
> Department of Nutrition and Food
> University of Massachusetts
> Amherst, Massachusetts 01002

BACKUP PROGRAMS

The six backup programs include the Technical Guidance Center for Environmental Quality, which assembles information and publishes a bulletin on environmental conditions; the Environmental Quality Executive Council of the College of Agriculture, which develops approaches to environmental problems; the Institute on Man and His Environment, which provides an interdisciplinary approach to environmental problems; the Water Resources Research Center; the Committee on Environmental Quality; and a proposed interdepartmental curriculum in Resource Development.

For further information, contact:

> Mrs. Ruth Kreplick
> Department of Environmental Sciences
> Technical Guidance Center for Environmental Quality

> Dr. W. J. Mellon
> College of Agriculture
> Environmental Quality Executive Council

> Dr. Carl Swanson
> Department of Botany
> Institute on Man and His Environment

> Dr. Bernard Berger
> Water Resources Research Center

> Dr. W. S. Motts
> Department of Geology
> Committee on Environmental Quality

> Dr. J. S. Larson
> Department of Forestry and Wildlife
> Interdepartmental curriculum

All correspondence to the above should be addressed in care of University of Massachusetts, Amherst, Massachusetts 01002.

McNEESE STATE UNIVERSITY
Lake Charles, Louisiana

WILDLIFE MANAGEMENT

The purpose of this curriculum is to prepare students for employment with the state and federal governments in areas related to wildlife conservation and management.

ENVIRONMENTAL SCIENCE

This curriculum is designed to provide the student with sufficient flexibility to move into many areas of endeavor. The degree in environmental science enables the individual to obtain a position in industry, in a private institution, or in a governmental agency; or, the degree holder may pursue graduate work in the same area or related field.

For further information, contact:

> Dr. Robert L. Bryant
> Department of Wildlife Management
> McNeese State University
> Lake Charles, Louisiana 70601

UNIVERSITY OF MICHIGAN, SCHOOL OF NATURAL RESOURCES
Ann Arbor, Michigan

The School of Natural Resources offers a broad undergraduate program in Natural Resources which provides flexibility for the student to pursue either a general curriculum with environmental and resource concentration, or within this framework, a more specific curriculum tailored to develop some professional competence in a specific natural resource.

ENVIRONMENTAL COMMUNICATION

The Environmental Communications option to the Environmental Education and Outdoor Recreation Program is designed to train students in the effective transfer of environmental information, primarily for the purpose of stimulating and fostering sound environmental action, and to evaluate the effect of the media on environmental and related social problems. The communicator, for example, may be required to translate complex scientific information into a form which can be understood by an intended audience, and to sensitize and motivate this audience to act on its knowledge.

All students who pursue this option will have in common (1) an understanding of environmental problems, their origins, and possible resolutions; (2) a sound knowledge of human behavior and the psychology of influence and motivation as it relates to the environmental issues; and (3) a command area to develop graduate courses, seminars and work-study programs for students in this and allied programs, and teach one undergraduate course annually for any students in the school who want an introduction to the theory and practice of Environmental Advocacy.

ENVIRONMENTAL ADVOCACY

Environmental Advocacy is an option to the Environmental Education and Outdoor Recreation Program which seeks to relate the needs of contemporary society to the policy decisions generated through environmental management. More specifically, the option is directed toward assuring that environmental decision-making results in equitable distribution of socio-economic costs and benefits. The major thrust of the program is to train individuals who will work with and for those who are least able to articulate environmental difficulties and who are least able to make the present socio-political system work as well for them as it can work for others of greater political efficacy. Within this philosophical framework, emphasis is upon these concerns as they relate to racial, ethnic, and economic groups who are most affected by, and least able to organize effective action to correct the environmental problems which they endure.

Students in this option are trained to determine the various social implications of environmental decision and to participate in the development and use of strategies to bring about socio-economic costs and benefits which are equitable to all. Individual specializations as, for example, in Resource or Welfare Economics, Environmental Policy, Environmental Law, Community Organization or Planned Change and Intervention Strategies, are developed substantially through the work-study experiences.

LIVING WITH THE EARTH

The purpose of this program is to introduce many "alternative life skills" useful in living in close ecological balance with the environment. The "environment" may be an organic garden, a homestead or a small community. Subjects to be studied will be food (plant and animal) production, storage, energy production (from sun and wind) and total recycling of everything possible.

For further information, contact:

School of Natural Resources
University of Michigan
Ann Arbor, Michigan 48104

MICHIGAN TECHNOLOGICAL UNIVERSITY
Houghton, Michigan

FORESTRY AND ENVIRONMENTAL STUDIES

Michigan Technological University's program in forestry is one of the most broad-gauge academic offerings at the University. It leans heavily on the sciences basic to forestry—mathematics to calculus, chemistry, physics and biology. After securing a strong background in the basic sciences—all of which are requisites to environmental quality development—the core curriculum stresses applications of these subjects. Forest Soils, Urban Problems, Recreation Land Management, Forest Management, Forest Ecology, Wildlife Ecology, Area Planning and Design are a few of the areas of specialization.

The university has a ten million-acre commercial forest, and a new $1.4 million forestry building.

Michigan Tech also has an Environmental Studies Curriculum that leads to a Bachelor of Science degree in Engineering.

For further information, contact:

Gene A. Hesterberg
Department of Forestry
Michigan Technological University
Houghton, Michigan 49931

MISSISSIPPI STATE UNIVERSITY
State College, Mississippi

ENVIRONMENTAL SCIENCE

Mississippi State has a program whereby a student can major in environmental science by choosing a general science curriculum. This curriculum requires 30 hours in a particular area of science and a total of 60 hours in scientific courses. Such a student may readily choose courses of an environmental nature once he has taken the elementary courses in the various departments. The Department of Zoology has an emphasis in natural history, and has courses in geology and other biological areas which are specifically directed toward ecological problems. In addition, students may take courses in the Department of Wildlife Management.

For further information, contact:

Mississippi State University
State College, Mississippi 39762

UNIVERSITY OF NEW HAMPSHIRE
Durham, New Hampshire

ENVIRONMENTAL MAJORS

The University of New Hampshire offers majors in:

(1) Environmental Conservation, giving a broad background in environmental problems;

(2) Resource Economics, offering training in resource economics, public resource policy, resource management, conservation economics, community resource development, and regional economics;

(3) Wildlife management.

For further information, contact:

University of New Hampshire
Durham, New Hampshire 03824

NEW MEXICO STATE UNIVERSITY
Las Cruces, New Mexico

WATER RESOURCES RESEARCH INSTITUTE

The basic mission of the Water Resources Research Institute is to plan and conduct basic and applied research on either single or interdisciplinary approach to complex water problems. Training is provided for scientists through research activities and experimentation.

Financed by federal, state, local and private funds, the institute carries on its broad program at New Mexico State and other New Mexico institutions through a program of support for faculty and graduate research projects.

For further information, contact:

New Mexico State University
Las Cruces, New Mexico 88001

THE CITY UNIVERSITY OF NEW YORK
New York, New York

ENVIRONMENTAL TECHNOLOGY

The City University of New York will offer a two-year environmental technology program. The course, intended to train pollution fighters, is expected to enroll about 30 students this year. Areas covered will be biology, chemistry, pollution monitoring, public health and pollution control.

For further information, contact:

City University of New York
535 E. 80th St.
New York, New York 10031

STATE UNIVERSITY OF NEW YORK AT ALBANY
Albany, New York

ENVIRONMENTAL STUDIES

At the time of this publication the university does not offer either a second field or major in environmentally-related courses or a sequence of such courses. University regulations give those students who do not have a mandated combined major-second-field the option of submitting individually developed interdisciplinary second fields to their major department for approval.

For further information, contact:

Mr. Louis Ismay
Associate Coordinator of Environmental Studies
State University of New York at Albany
1400 Washington Avenue
Albany, New York 12203

STATE UNIVERSITY OF NEW YORK AT BINGHAMTON
Binghamton, New York

BIOLOGICAL SCIENCES

State University of New York at Binghamton does not have a formal program in which a student can enroll as a major in environmental sciences. However, they do offer all the requirements for such a degree.

As a major in Biological Sciences, a student may decide

to substitute geology, geography, anthropology, and other related disciplines for the major requirements. Biological sciences, geology and geography have quite a few joint projects in environmental sciences from which the student can benefit. As a result, the student can design a tailormade program depending on which area of environmental sciences he wishes to concentrate. The university feels that a definite prescribed program is not *pedagogically* sound since the area of environmental sciences is so broad.

Another route a student may take is to apply to the Innovational Projects board with a program of his own design. If approved, the student can graduate in any multidiscipline area he chooses.

For further information, contact:

Roger H. Trumbore
Associate Professor and Chairman
Department of Biological Sciences
State University of New York at Binghamton
Binghamton, New York 13901

STATE UNIVERSITY OF NEW YORK AT STONY BROOK
Stony Brook, New York

ENVIRONMENTAL STUDIES

The interdisciplinary program in environmental studies (ENS) is designed to provide students with a basic understanding of man's interdependence with his environment and to prepare them to take part as informed citizens in environmental planning. The program can serve as the basic preparation for students intending to pursue professional studies in any of a variety of fields dealing with problems of the environment. In addition to taking a core sequence of courses, each student will be expected to begin developing competence in a specialty and gain some practice in applying it to environmental problems as a member of an interdisciplinary team. Courses for the specialty requirement may be satisfied by completing a regular departmental major with an emphasis on courses relevant to environmental studies.

For further information, contact:

State University of New York at Stony Brook
Stony Brook, New York 11790

NORTHLAND COLLEGE
Ashland, Wisconsin

ENVIRONMENTAL STUDIES PROGRAM

This program is broad and interdisciplinary in scope and the people who major in the program have a great deal of latitude in the courses they may choose to complete the major.

The primary objectives of this program are:

(1) To aid students in acquiring the basic understanding that man is an inseparable part of his environment-system which consists of man, society, and the biophysical setting and that man can change the interrelationships of the environment-system.

(2) To aid students in acquiring an understanding of the biophysical environment, both man-made and natural.

(3) To aid students in understanding problems of the biophysical setting that confronts man, how the problems can be solved, and the responsibility of man to work for their solutions.

For further information, contact:

> Bruce Alan Goety, Chairman
> Environmental Studies Committee
> Northland College
> Ashland, Wisconsin 54806

NORTHWESTERN STATE COLLEGE
Alva, Oklahoma

AGECOLOGY

This new program at Northwestern State College in AgEcology will train specialists with a knowledge of the interrelationships between agricultural practices and the natural ecosystems.

For further information, contact:

> Department of AgEcology
> Northwestern State College
> Alva, Oklahoma 73717

NORWICH UNIVERSITY
Northfield, Vermont

ENVIRONMENTAL TECHNOLOGY

Aided by a grant from the National Science Foundation, Norwich has instituted an innovative four-year curriculum in Environmental Technology. The purpose of the curriculum is to educate and train environmental specialists of the future.

Because the environmental technologist must have a strong background in many areas of understanding, the Norwich program covers a wide range of studies and "hands-on" training. The research and study takes the students far beyond the classroom.

They are brought into direct contact with environmental problems by working and conferring with key personnel in governmental agencies and laboratories, by studying industrial plants and recycling units, and by carrying out individual projects in their own areas of interest.

The students also learn to preserve natural beauty through esthetic environmental planning and programming.

The Environmental Technology program, which is interdisciplinary in nature, involves many departments of the University, including civil, mechanical, and electrical engineering, physics, biology, and chemistry.

For more information, contact:

Director of Admissions
Norwich University
Northfield, Vermont 05663

OHIO UNIVERSITY
Athens, Ohio

BACHELOR OF GENERAL STUDIES

At this time Ohio University does not offer a multidisciplinary major in environmental sciences. They do offer a student-designed degree, the Bachelor of General Studies, which could be easily fitted to environmental studies. The only requirements for the Bachelor of General Studies are 180 quarter hours, 90 of which must be upper-division courses. Courses could be selected from geology (which offers a separate major in water conservation), engineering, botany, and zoology to provide a fairly comprehensive program in environmental studies.

For further information, contact:

> University College of Ohio University
> Chubb Hall
> Athens, Ohio 45701

THE UNIVERSITY OF OKLAHOMA
Norman, Oklahoma

MULTIDISCIPLINARY PROGRAMS

The University of Oklahoma has two cooperating, multidisciplinary, environmentally-oriented programs:

The program in Environmental Science is a division of the Civil Engineering School in the College of Engineering.

The College of Environmental Design is "horizontally administered" college which seeks to encourage and coordinate multidisciplinary environmental activities and programs of all kinds throughout the University.

For further information, contact:

> College of Environmental Design
> The University of Oklahoma
> Norman, Oklahoma 73069

OLIVET COLLEGE
Olivet, Michigan

INTERDISCIPLINARY STUDIES

Olivet College does not have a formal Environmental Science major. However, through their interdisciplinary studies program, the Olivet student may select an "interest major," rather than a departmental major. By this route, the student and his adviser plan a course of interdisciplinary study, aiming toward a specific type of preparation. "Environmental Science" is certainly one of the possibilities.

For further information, contact:

> John M. Roberts, Ph.D.
> Professor, Interdisciplinary Studies
> Olivet College
> Olivet, Michigan 49076

UNIVERSITY OF OREGON
Charleston, Oregon

INSTITUTE OF MARINE BIOLOGY

The University of Oregon's Institute of Marine Biology offers several programs that study environmental problems. An Undergraduate Research Participant program, sponsored by the National Science Foundation, places about seven students into field work each summer. Its Student Originated Studies program, also sponsored by the NSF, allows students to probe more deeply into problems encountered in the Research Participant program.

Also offered is an Environmental Projects course, emphasizing biology and land use planning; and recently instituted is a multidisciplinary Environmental Studies curriculum including courses in biology, sociology, geography and architecture. The institute expects to expand this program into a full-year offering.

For further information, contact:

Paul P. Rudy, Director
Oregon Institute of Marine Biology
University of Oregon
Charleston, Oregon 97420

THE PENNSYLVANIA STATE UNIVERSITY
University Park, Pennsylvania

ENVIRONMENTAL SCIENCE

Penn State has two multidisciplinary environmental science majors at the undergraduate level. They are:

Environmental Resource Management, College of Agriculture

Dr. Russell J. Hutnik, Chairman, 312 Forest Resource Lab, University Park, Pa. 16802

Environmental Protection Engineering, College of Engineering

Dr. John Nesbitt, Chairman, 116 Sackett, University Park, Pa. 16802

For further information, contact the respective chairman.

PITZER COLLEGE
Member of the Claremont Colleges
Claremont, California

ENVIRONMENTAL STUDIES

Environmental studies is an interdisciplinary program drawing upon the resources of all the Claremont Colleges.

Students are expected to plan their programs in close consultation with an environmental studies advisor, and to complete satisfactorily at least 10 courses chosen so as to include introductory and advanced work.

Students must also undertake fieldwork, or an internship, or an action project, either in connection with a course, or as independent study, or in conjunction with the senior seminar, Environmental Studies 190, is required of all seniors. Exceptional students may be invited to undertake an honors thesis in the senior year.

For further information, contact:

Mr. Rodman
Pitzer College
Member of the Claremont Colleges
Claremont, California 91711

PRINCETON UNIVERSITY
Princeton, New Jersey

COUNCIL ON ENVIRONMENTAL STUDIES

The Council on Environmental Studies is charged with the coordination of teaching and research programs in environmental science, technology and planning. Undergraduate students prepare for environmental careers or advanced study by supplementing normal programs in their own departments with planned selections from courses in other departments. Independent work may be pursued under the direction of faculty members throughout the university whose interests lie in the environmental area. In addition, the Council places special emphasis on the fostering and funding of interdisciplinary graduate programs including those with strong inputs from the social sciences.

For further information, contact:

Princeton University
Princeton, New Jersey 08540

PURDUE UNIVERSITY
Lafayette, Indiana

ENVIRONMENTAL HEALTH

The Environmental Health Program at Purdue University is a coherent, but extremely flexible, interdisciplinary program geared to meet the individual needs and interests of each student. Each student will work closely with a member of the faculty who will be his counselor, to formulate an individual plan of study to meet the students specific educational objectives.

For further information, contact:

> John E. Christian, Director
> Institute for Environmental Health
> Purdue University
> Lafayette, Indiana 47907

REGIS COLLEGE
Denver, Colorado

ENVIRONMENTAL BIOLOGY

Regis offers a variety of courses under the concentration Environmental Biology, including general biology, general ecology, human ecology and population dynamics. Field work is required.

For further information, contact:

> Regis College
> 3539 West 50th Avenue Parkway
> Denver, Colorado 80221

RENSSELAER POLYTECHNIC INSTITUTE
Troy, New York

ENVIRONMENTAL ENGINEERING

Rensselaer's program in Environmental Engineering is offered to students on three levels: bachelor's, master's, and doctoral. All three levels provide an unusual opportunity for the qualified students to prepare for a career in this expanding area of practice. The program provides an outstanding opportunity for the creative student who is willing to deal with interesting problems of vital concern as well as community health and wellbeing.

The Environmental Engineering Curriculum is subdivided into five major fields: (1) air pollution; (2) water resources, including water supply and wastewater treatment, (3) solid wastes; (4) radiological health; and (5) noise abatement.

For further information, contact:

Dr. Ray W. Shade
Chairman, Environmental Engineering Curriculum
Rensselaer Polytechnic Institute
Troy, New York 12181

RUTGERS UNIVERSITY
New Brunswick, New Jersey

AGRICULTURE & ENVIRONMENTAL SCIENCE

Curricula in Agriculture and Environmental Science are designed to provide students with liberal education and specialized and professional instruction in agriculture and the environmental sciences. The eight core curricula offered will prepare men and women for plant and animal production, for teaching and research professions, or for one of the numerous businesses related to the fields of agriculture and certain of the other applied biological and environmental sciences. About 5 percent of the graduates become producers of agricultural commodities; 30-50 percent go to graduate schools to prepare for careers in teaching, research, or some other scientific occupation related to plants, animals, and the environment; and the remainder accept employment in one or another of the phases of business related to agriculture and the environmental sciences.

The program for the freshman year includes courses in biology, chemistry, English, mathematics, plant and animal sciences for all four-year curricula. Beginning with the sophomore year the student, with faculty guidance and approval, pursues one of eight core curricula: Animal Science, Agricultural Science, Plant Science, Preparation for Research, Agricultural Business, Food Science, Landscape Architecture, and Environmental Science. The student has the choice between pursuing broad general programs with a wide selection of elective subjects or a more specific program (major) where the choice of elective subjects is based upon a career objective. The specific programs are indicated after the title of the core curriculum under which the program is usually developed.

For further information, contact:

Rutgers University
New Brunswick, New Jersey 08903

SACRAMENTO STATE COLLEGE
Sacramento, California

ENVIRONMENTAL STUDIES

Sacramento State College intends to arm the successful student with tools, so that when he is considering possible solutions to a planetary problem, he can better decide (1) how many people are going to be affected? (2) for how long? (3) at what level of culture? and (4) what are the chances of backing out if things go wrong? Sacramento State expects the student to learn to treat these as an interdependent set, as indeed they are.

Course work, research and individual projects make up the curriculum. Though many units are required for this major (58-63), by carefully choosing general education courses to satisfy pre-requisites, there is no undue stress on a student to finish his degree in the usual length of time.

GENERAL EDUCATION PROGRAM

Students will be required to take 46 units of General Education. The students matriculating at SSC should plan this curriculum so as to choose those G.E. courses which are most related to Environmental Studies and which can be used as prerequisites for those courses which can be applied to the major in Environmental Studies or to the student's required minor.

For further information, contact:

Wes Jackson
Environmental Studies, Chairman
Sacramento State College
6000 Jay Street
Sacramento, California 95819

SAN JOSE STATE COLLEGE
San Jose, California

ENVIRONMENTAL STUDIES

Boring lectures, afternoons in the library, philosophical discussions. That may be the norm for most college students, but not for many in the Environmental Studies Department at San Jose State College.

Half of the courses offered by this department involve environmental activism rather than straight book learning and exams.

Dr. Donald W. Aitken, conservation activist and former astrophysics researcher at Stanford University, heads the department. He is a founding director of Friends of the Earth and is scientific coordinator for the John Muir Institute of Environmental Studies.

According to Dr. Aitken, the department grew out of the mass volunteer effort students have made during the past in working for various environmental groups. "We are providing a structure for the same kinds of things," he said. "We're taking environmental activism and seeing if we can build it into a whole educational process."

In a recycling course, students assess the practical economics and current possibilities for recycling of natural resources. They have put their ideas into practice with the establishment of a campus recycling center. The center, manned by the students in the class, has two purposes. The first is to change attitudes and secondly they must show the city that recycling is feasible.

The students hope to convince the city that it can save money in garbage collection by having solid items sorted out and recycled. John T. Stanley, biology lecturer and adviser for the center, said that if enough people want to recycle, scavenger companies will get on the bandwagon and buy reusable waste, thus lowering the cost of city collections.

Reaction to the center has been tremendous. A small one-room cottage that is the home of the center has long been overflowing with goods to be sent to plants for recycling. The class members are looking for a larger building to accommodate the influx of materials. The center receives waste products from dormitories, student housing, and from others in the campus community. It receives 15 to 20 calls a day from people outside the college community who want to know where they can bring their recyclable goods.

In a conservation course offered last year, students were graded on their efforts to solve a conservation problem. "For many of them, they felt for the first time that they could fight in the system. They found that they could work with the government, for the government could work for them," Stanley said. He explained that one of the students was disappointed because the government took over his project. The problem only had to be pointed out to the government agency to set it in action.

Another course designed to foster interaction between the campus and the community is an environmental information center. "It is an attempt to provide information about environmental issues," Stanley, said. "It is providing a service that is not available elsewhere." He started the center last year in response to the paucity of environmental information. Stanley was then Director of Education and Information for the San Jose State Environmental Studies Institute, which has become the research subdivision of the new department.

This year the center is completely run by students taking the course. In addition to enlarging the library, they have started a speakers' bureau. The students and instructors go out into the community and speak to groups when invited.

The center also gathers information for teachers on getting environmental films for classes. In addition, it produces a calendar of environmental events, and the students exchange ideas with conservation groups.

Still another activist class is an environmental films and film-making class. Dr. Aitken originally planned to have the class evaluate films this semester to determine what films are still needed. He hoped to obtain equipment next semester for the students to actually make their own environmental films.

"Everything that is being done in environmental education today is an experiment. People who are doing it must understand that you are doing things differently when you are experimenting with something than when you are instituting something in its finished form. We will continue to experiment with courses for an environmental studies major for two years, after which we hope to define the most useful curriculum that we are searching for."

For further information, contact:

San Jose State College
San Jose, California 95112

The degree program in Environmental Studies has been developed around sufficient flexibility and diversity of options so that the student may tailor his own program in accordance with his own interests, skills and goals; and it has been structured to encourage off-campus activities and internships in public service.

The educational program in Environmental Studies is aimed at imparting useful comprehension in four broad areas:

(1) The Natural Biophysical Environment
(2) The Man-Altered Environment
(3) Man's Perception of his Environment
(4) Tools and Techniques

Accordingly, the entire program of core curricula and electives has been conceived to provide a balanced introduction to all four areas, rather than to specific disciplines, but with a major emphasis directing the student toward a chosen specialty.

B. A. IN ENVIRONMENTAL STUDIES WITH A MAJOR CONCENTRATION IN THE SOCIAL SCIENCES AND HUMANITIES

This degree consists of a concentration in an area relevant to Environmental Studies centered in the Social Sciences or Humanities. This concentration is balanced by a required greater depth in the environmental sciences.

B. A. IN ENVIRONMENTAL STUDIES WITH A MAJOR CONCENTRATION IN THE NATURAL SCIENCES

This degree consists of a concentration in an area of Environmental Science, with the aim of leading toward advanced work or a useful specialty.

B. S. IN ENVIRONMENTAL STUDIES WITH A MAJOR CONCENTRATION IN ENVIRONMENTAL TECHNOLOGY OR MANAGEMENT

This degree consists of a concentration in a technical specialty aimed at careers presently in demand or projected to be in demand in environmental industry monitoring, protection or control, or as the basis for further undergraduate or graduate work in that specialty.

For further information, contact:

> Donald Aitken, Chairman
> Department of Environmental Studies
> San Jose State College
> San Jose, California 95114

UNIVERSITY OF SOUTHERN MISSISSIPPI
Hattiesburg, Mississippi

ENVIRONMENTAL SCIENCE

The newly instituted Environmental Science program at the University of Southern Mississippi adds a new dimension of relevance to the university's academic program. The program has made students in all fields aware of pressing environmental problems, possible solutions to these problems, and ways of bringing about results through the application of their own specialty.

The interdisciplinary major leading to a degree in environmental science draws heavily on courses in biology, chemistry, geology, and physics. The major is bolstered by a freshman course, Basic Environmental Studies, which takes advantage of the better scientific training of entering students. The curriculum centers around three senior courses—Pollution Detection, Pollution Control, and Electronics for Scientists—and is rounded out by meteorology, environmental geology and courses in computer sciences.

Recently an Institute of Environmental Science was organized at the University of Southern Mississippi to provide an outlet for the skills of environmentally oriented scientists and students. The skills of these students are also utilized on the many field trips sponsored by the department.

For further information, contact:

Dr. Charles R. Brent
Director of Environmental Studies
Southern Station, Box 314
Hattiesburg, Mississippi 39401

STANFORD UNIVERSITY
Stanford, California

*ENVIRONMENTAL ENGINEERING, URBAN
PLANNING AND OCEAN ENGINEERING*

Students at Stanford may major in Environmental Engineering by gaining approval of their programs by the Undergraduate Council. The students will be included in the broad areas of Applied Science and Engineering Science and can specialize in Environmental Engineering, Urban Planning, or Ocean Engineering if the programs they design meet with the Council's approval.

For further information, contact:

Stanford University
Stanford, California 94305

ST. EDWARDS UNIVERSITY
Austin, Texas

ENVIRONMENTAL STUDIES

This program consists of an interdisciplinary major proposed for students interested in the study of the environment: physical, biological, and human, for the purpose of gaining an understanding of modern man's environment from a holistic point of view. The program of studies will not focus on the solution of particular environmental problems, but on providing an insight into the complex nature of man's environment, the methods used to acquire a better understanding of it, and the lines of action designed to prevent its deterioration and possibly improve it.

The student is advised to take a concentration of electives in the area in which he would like to work as an environmentalist. The idea is to provide the student with a broad overview of modern man's environment and at the same time enough information in one area to let him get into environmental work on a professional basis.

In the fall of 1971 Saint Edwards University opened an Environics Center. The Center is oriented toward both the Austin and the St. Edwards communities.

For further information, contact:

St. Edwards University
3101 S. Congress Avenue
Austin, Texas 78704

ST. LOUIS UNIVERSITY
St. Louis, Missouri

ENVIRONMENTAL STUDIES

St. Louis University offers, through its Institute of Environmental Studies, a program leading to a certificate in environmental studies. The Institute of Environmental Studies sponsors problem-oriented teaching and research in an interdisciplinary context which explicitly recognizes the complexity of environmental problems. The certificate program is intended to enable the student to identify and understand environmental problem areas in order that he may be able to apply the skills of his area of concentration to the special problem-complex.

The certificate program is based on the belief that environmental problems involve all aspects of man's biological, psychological and cultural life. The program is interdisciplinary, including the natural sciences, the social sciences and the humanities. It is designed to furnish the student with an integrative focus for undergraduate study, by providing a knowledge base in the various disciplines as well as a sense of organic relatedness of man and his environment.

For further information, write to:

St. Louis University
Institute of Environmental Studies
221 N. Grand Blvd.
St. Louis, Missouri 63103

SAN DIEGO STATE UNIVERSITY
San Diego, California

ENVIRONMENTAL HEALTH
San Diego State College offers a major in Environmental Health. This major is offered by the department of Microbiology and includes courses in Microbiology, Zoology, Biology, Health Science and Safety, Public Administration and Engineering.

For further information, contact:

> San Diego State College
> 5402 College Avenue
> San Diego, California 92115

SANGAMON STATE UNIVERSITY
Springfield, Illinois

MULTIDISCIPLINARY STUDY
Sangamon State University does not maintain a program in the science area but it does offer students the opportunity to pursue a multi-disciplinary course of study which leads to a B.A. in Environments and People. This program is tailored to the individual student's needs and goals.

The students at Sangamon have organized an Environmental Activists Club and are currently engaged in several recycling projects.

For further information, contact:

> Walter D. Johnson
> Sangamon State University
> Springfield, Illinois 62703

SEATTLE UNIVERSITY
Seattle, Washington

ENVIRONMENTAL STUDIES
Seattle University has programs in Environmental Studies.

For further information, contact:

> D. W. Schroeder, Ph.D.
> Dean
> School of Science and Engineering
> Seattle University
> Seattle, Washington 98122

SLIPPERY ROCK STATE COLLEGE
Slippery Rock, Pennsylvania

ENVIRONMENTAL SCIENCES

Slippery Rock State College initiated the first comprehensive undergraduate study in Environmental Sciences in the Commonwealth of Pennsylvania. The objectives of this study are:

(1) To provide the student with intellectual stimulus and knowledge of environmental interrelationships, so that he may be a critical observer in a complex socioeconomic society that must use its environment intelligently.

(2) To prepare young environmental scientists for technical and administrative positions in city health departments, planning commissions, industries, and state and federal environmental agencies.

(3) To equip students for graduate studies in environmental sciences.

For further information, contact:

J. W. Shiner, Chairman
Recreation Department
Slippery Rock State College
Slippery Rock, Pennsylvania 16057

SOUTHAMPTON COLLEGE
Southampton, New York

ENVIRONMENTAL STUDIES

The requirement for a degree in Environmental Studies at Southampton consists of four parts: the core, the concentration, the thesis, and participation in the Environmental Center. These requirements should be considered as guidelines which will normally be followed. Minor changes can be made, in individual cases, for good and sufficient reason, with the approval of the Planning Committee.

The Core consists of sixteen courses so distributed as to give the student a broad base in environmentally related areas of natural science, social science, and humanities.

The Concentration consists of six courses centering around an area of Natural Science, Social Science, Administration, or Humanistic Studies. For a student concentrating in an area of Natural Science, Social Science, or Humanistic Studies, the concentration will consist of six courses selected by the student and approved by an advisory committee consisting of at least two faculty members.

The idea of an undergraduate thesis is central to Southampton's notion of what an environmental studies program should be. It is important to get out of the classroom and into the real world as soon and as often as possible. The student will select, plan, carry out, and report on a project in an environmentally-related area. He will work with one or more faculty members and may involve lower-level students as associates. Credit for the thesis equivalent to one, one and one-half, or two courses will be given.

In order to gain practical experience in working on environmental problems, to gain an activist outlook, and to prepare for tackling a thesis project, the study is required to participate actively in the Environmental Center at least one semester for each year that he is at Southampton College. Determination of what constitutes active participation is left to the Planning Committee. Evaluation of the extent of each student's participation will be done, mainly, by the student himself.

Students will be admitted to the program provisionally on entering the College. Toward the end of the sophomore year, they will formally reappraise their commitment as Environmental Studies majors. Their decision will be made as much on the basis of attitude, activity and interest as upon grades. The purpose of this provision is to provide encouragement rather than mere evaluation, and is not intended as an elitist screening-out process. For students in good standing, the decision to remain in the program or to leave will be their own.

For at least the first year, the student will have at least two advisors representing at least two divisions of the college. After the student selects a field of concentration, he or she will be advised by the division of his or her chosen field.

All students who so desire will be assisted in finding significant off-campus internships or work study programs appropriate to their goals during one or more short semesters or summers.

For further information, contact:

John W. Andrews
The Environmental Center at Southampton College
Southampton, New York 11968

SOUTHEASTERN MASSACHUSETTS UNIVERSITY
North Dartmouth, Massachusetts

ENVIRONMENTAL STUDIES

The environment-related studies at Southeastern Massachusetts University are centered in curricula developed by the faculties of biology and engineering and focus largely on courses and research related to coastal zone environment.

The Biology Department offers an undergraduate option in marine science leading to a baccalaureate degree and the Engineering Department offers several undergraduate options in Ocean Engineering, with special emphasis on electrical engineering in the ocean environment.

This university has extensive controlled environment facilities in their new research building, and has a 65 foot research vessel RV Corsair which is used extensively for instructional purposes. The 730 acre campus includes pond, bog, woodland and open field environments which are used for teaching and experimental purposes. A 20-acre waterfront site on nearby Gooseberry Island provides dune and intertidal sites for environmental studies.

For further information, contact:

John J. Reardon
Professor and Chairman of Biology
Southeastern Massachusetts University
North Dartmouth, Massachusetts 02747

SOUTHERN ILLINOIS UNIVERSITY DEPARTMENT OF FORESTRY
Carbondale, Illinois

FOREST RESOURCE MANAGEMENT

Forest Resource Management includes instruction in forest production, multiple-use resource management, wood utilization science, and specialized courses in forest recreation planning and development. This specialization includes the ten areas of study in the forestry curriculum recommendations of the Society of American Foresters. Outdoor Recreation Resource Management provides training for management of the nation's outdoor recreation heritage. The courses offered are among those recommended by the National Parks and Recreation Association. One spring quarter of practical field courses is required. During this period, students live in the field and pay living expenses involved. The recreation management student does not attend field camp, but instead travels through selected sections of the United States on a three-week field tour of outdoor recreation and park facilities in late August and early September.

For further information, contact:

Department of Forestry
Southern Illinois University
Carbondale, Illinois 62901

SOUTHERN OREGON COLLEGE
Ashland, Oregon

GENERAL STUDIES

The curriculum at Southern Oregon College is so structured that students who do not wish to major in a specific area (such as Chemistry or English or History or Psychology, etc.) may take a major in General Studies.

There are two options under the General Studies degree: A divisional major in one of the broad areas (Humanities, or Science Mathematics or Social Science), or interdisciplinary majors which allow students to put together a major across divisional lines combining work from two to four subject fields. These General Studies majors would permit students to develop a multi-disciplinary major in Environmental Science.

For further information, contact:

Arthur Kreisman
Dean of Arts and Sciences
Southern Oregon College
Ashland, Oregon 97520

SPRINGFIELD COLLEGE
Springfield, Massachusetts

ENVIRONMENTAL STUDIES

An undergraduate program in Environmental Studies has been prepared for students concerned with the human habitat and wishing to pursue careers dedicated to helping improve it—a human service too long neglected. The program makes possible many patterns of study by synchronizing arts and sciences so that they can mesh meaningfully with professional studies in education, community affairs, recreation, health, and physical education for ecologically sensitive learning, living and leisure. Emphasis is on the balance between the artificial and the natural in emerging life-styles to help The Whole Man in a Wholesome World.

For further information, contact:

Dean of Admissions
Springfield College
Springfield, Massachusetts 01109

STATE UNIVERSITY COLLEGE AT BUFFALO
Buffalo, New York

ENVIRONMENTAL SCIENCES

The Environmental Sciences Curriculum is primarily designed to enable students who have majored in environmental (health) science at a two-year college to transfer, with minimal loss of credits, to Buffalo State where they can either earn a bachelor's degree in Biology or Chemistry while continuing to specialize in environmental sciences. Therefore, a graduate of this program will have training in breadth as well as depth.

Instruction of ES courses will be provided by members of the Biology and Chemistry faculties as well as the staff of the Great Lakes Laboratory.

Facilities of the Laboratory include a field station on Lake Erie (seven minutes from the Buffalo State campus), four research vessels, including a 66-foot T-boat that has been fully modified for Lake Erie pollution investigations and one of the most complete libraries of current material on water pollution. Opportunities for participation such as part-time and summer employment in the GLL's sponsored research, which amounts to over $100,000 per year, will be available to students in the program.

For further information, contact:

Dr. Robert A. Sweeney, Director
Great Lakes Laboratory
State University College
5 Porter Avenue
Buffalo, New York 14201
Telephone No. (716) 862-5422

STEPHENS COLLEGE
Columbia, Missouri
PROGRAM IN ENVIRONMENTAL SCIENCE

The program in Environmental Science at Stephens College is designed to produce a highly qualified individual for work in governmental, educational or industrial environmental sciences.

Stephens College has an Environmental Action Group active on its campus. The club has been established since the fall term of 1969. The club is involved with a recycling program on campus. The club also has an education lab on campus, political action groups, fund raising for Missouri Nature Conservancy, population education programs and county removal programs.

Along with numerous campus activities to supplement their program, the college publishes two environmentally-centered publications: *Guide for Environmental Action* and *Bounty News*.

For further information, write to:

H. Charles Laun
Biology Department
Stephens College Post Office
Columbia, Missouri 65201

SYRACUSE UNIVERSITY
Syracuse, New York
ENVIRONMENTAL ENGINEERING

An interdisciplinary committee composed of eight faculty representatives of the various departments of engineering establishes the guidelines for the specific degrees in environmental engineering. Each student is encouraged to develop an individual program of study which he feels will best lead to his educational goals, and he will be assisted in this effort by a faculty adviser from the environmental engineering committee. Before the end of the freshman year, the student submits a tentative written proposal for his four-year program of study to the committee for approval. This proposal may subsequently be altered to meet any change in the career objectives of the student.

For further information, contact:

> Dr. Nelson L. Nemerow, Chairman
> Environmental Engineering Faculty Advisory
>   Committee
> Hinds Hall
> Syracuse University
> Syracuse, New York 13210

TABOR COLLEGE
Hillsboro, Kansas

SOCIAL WORK AND BIOLOGY-ECOLOGY

The social work program at Tabor College is especially unique for a small college. This college is working on programs which will allow students to major in social work in minor biology with an emphasis on ecology.

The smallness of this institution allows them to couple the environmental aspect to any human service related major. Courses in biology would include basic biological science, zoology, botany and ecology as the core environmental science curriculum for an environmental emphasis attached to any major.

Tabor is also working towards plans to develop an environmental science major to go along with the service oriented philosophy of the college. The Environmental Science major would include the above courses plus courses in chemistry such as quantitative analysis, organic chemistry or biochemistry. There is considerable flexibility in the approach that will allow Tabor to tailor a program to each individual student. For instance, a student may want to include some medical courses in his curriculum as part of his

environmental science major or minor. These courses might be human anatomy and physiology or general physiology.
For further information, contact:

> Department of Biology
> Tabor College
> Hillsboro, Kansas 67063

TEMPLE UNIVERSITY
Philadelphia, Pennsylvania

ENVIRONMENTAL TECHNOLOGY

The Temple University Technical Institute has developed a program in Environmental Technology to prepare young people for careers in the environmental control field. This is a two-year program which is designed to give the student a strong background in the basic sciences, an introduction to both the techniques of environmental measurements and environmental control.
For further information, contact:

> Temple University Technical Institute
> Broad and Montgomery Avenue
> Philadelphia, Pennsylvania 19122

TRINITY COLLEGE
Hartford, Connecticut

URBAN-ENVIRONMENTAL STUDIES

The Urban-Environmental Studies Program at Trinity does not consist of very much in terms of specific courses scheduled for the year. It does consist of some very good course experiments, an active Community Affairs and Open Semester program, and an institutional flexibility which will permit students to pursue a wide variety of urban and environmental interests. What is offered is a plan for the future development of the program, and should be thought of as a basis for discussion rather than a fixed and immutable program.

The U-E Program is composed of the following elements: a one-year introductory course, a group of basic sophomore courses, junior and senior seminars, an urban internship and accompanying seminar, and senior research. In addition we will require the student to emphasize some disciplinary concentration which constitutes the core of a traditional major and to choose a "theme" to guide his elective course selection in U-E Studies.

For further information, contact:

Andrew J. Gold, Director
Urban-Environmental Studies Program
Trinity College
Hartford, Connecticut 06106

THE UNITED STATES NAVAL ACADEMY
Annapolis, Maryland
DEPARTMENT OF ENVIRONMENTAL SCIENCES, OCEANOGRAPHY MAJOR

Oceanography is an inter-disciplinary science major involving the study of chemistry, physics, biology, and geology as they relate to our ocean environment and the effects of that environment on naval operations.

The oceanography major is a laboratory-oriented program with the most modern facilities including its own oceanographic vessel, a weather station and radiosonde system for study of the atmosphere, plus a wave tank, tide gauges, marine culture systems, and fully equipped laboratories.

For further information, contact:

The United States Naval Academy
Annapolis, Maryland 21402

UTAH STATE UNIVERSITY
Logan, Utah
ENVIRONMENT AND MAN

Utah State University is running an Environment and Man program which will seek to develop long-term concern over environmental problems in both students and instructors. By seeking to gain their objectives over time, the people involved in the program hope to promote sustained efforts to solve environmental problems and offset the public's proclivity for following headlines.

Environment and Man, which is administered primarily through the university's Division of Research, works as follows:

• A Director and a Steering Committee work as a team to evaluate environmental problems of the region and to stimulate and coordinate the development of task forces, colloquia and interdisciplinary research proposals.

• Task forces composed of faculty members and graduate students carry out such short-term projects as preparing research proposals, doing applied research, planning colloquia, recommending legislative action or suggesting action by public or private agencies.

• Colloquia involving faculty, students and people from other walks of life critically evaluate the available knowledge and recommend ways to solve problems.

• Interdisciplinary research proposals may be generated by the task forces or colloquia.

Currently, interdisciplinary research and colloquia programs under way or planned include: Waste Management, Land Use Planning, Environmental Education and Population Impacts on Environmental Quality.

For more information, contact:

Dr. C. M. McKell, Director
Room 225
Agricultural Sciences Bldg.
Utah State University
Logan, Utah 84321

WASHINGTON STATE UNIVERSITY
Pullman, Washington

ENVIRONMENTAL SCIENCE

The Program in Environmental Science at Washington State University includes cooperating members from departments in the colleges of Agriculture, Engineering, and Sciences and Arts. The course of study leads to the degrees of Bachelor of Sciences in Environmental Science and Master of Science in Environmental Science.

Through the program, students acquire an extensive background and a broad perspective that prepares them for a variety of roles in the study and management of the environment and its specific resources. Training in depth is obtained within any one of six optional areas of specialization: agriculture ecology, biological science, cultural ecology, environmental health, natural resources, and physical science.

A university-owned biological field study area (800 acres), located within 11 miles of the university campus, is available for graduate student research projects, and many agricultural experiment stations exist within the state. Also, facilities for air, water and land studies are provided by the Environmental and Sanitary Engineering Laboratories, the Water Research Center, and the Air Pollution Research Laboratory of the College of Engineering.

Requests for further information and applications, contact:

> Chairman
> Program in Environmental Science
> Washington State University
> Pullman, Washington 99163

WEST GEORGIA COLLEGE
Carrollton, Georgia

ENVIRONMENTAL STUDIES

Environmental Studies at West Georgia College has been established to achieve the following goals:

(1) To establish a minor program of study in environmental sciences so any student can gain a solid, occupationally useful but non-restrictive background in this field.

(2) To develop an academic awareness of basic environmental principles for all students.

(3) To develop a program of continuing education through classes and through the mass media so that the citizens of our region can comprehend a vital and rapidly changing field.

(4) To encourage research on the environment of the Northwest Georgia region so the college can meet both its academic obligation to the development of knowledge nationally and also meet its good

175

citizenship obligations for meaningful involvement in this region.

(5) To develop an environmental information collection and distribution center in cooperation with government and private agencies throughout the region.

For further information contact:

Charles D. Masters
West Georgia College
Carrollton, Georgia 30117

WESTMAN COLLEGE
Lemars, Iowa

ENVIRONMENTAL SCIENCE

Westman College offers a major in Environmental Science.

For further information, contact:

Wayne S. Marty
Director of Natural Sciences
Westman College
Lemars, Iowa 51031

WHITMAN COLLEGE
Walla Walla, Washington

ENVIRONMENTAL SCIENCE

Whitman offers four areas of concentration in its Environmental Science curriculum: sociology, economics, biology and chemistry. Background courses in environmental analysis; chemistry, general biology, or general zoology and botany; physiography of North America; principles of economics; and population are required. Other courses depend on the area of concentration, and seminars and directed independent study are available.

For further information, contact:

Whitman College
Walla Walla, Washington 99362

WILLAMETTE UNIVERSITY
Salem, Oregon

ENVIRONMENTAL SCIENCE

An Environmental Science Program is offered at Willamette University.

For further information, contact:

Williamette University
Salem, Oregon 97301

WILLIAMS COLLEGE
Williamstown, Massachusetts

CENTER FOR ENVIRONMENTAL STUDIES

The Center for Environmental Studies at Williams College has three basic objectives which it pursues both independently and in cooperation with the academic standards of the College:

(1) To provide a focal point for undergraduate teaching and faculty research in the environmental field.

(2) To relate the academic resources of Williams College to the planning and development needs of the surrounding region.

(3) To build a body of factual knowledge and professional understanding of the environmental issues developing in the metropolitan hinterland regions of the nation.

Research is being conducted near the campus on the forest ecology and land use history of an experimental forest near the campus, and on the effects of pollution abatement in the Hoosic River. The center has supported the Berkshire Panel on the Public Environment, is cooperating in an effort to improve environmental education in the elementary schools and the secondary schools in Berkshire County, Massachusetts, and has joined with the Berkshire County Regional Planning Commission on a study of the siting of electric power facilities.

For further information, contact:

> Williams College
> Center for Environmental Studies
> Williamstown, Massachusetts 01267

THE UNIVERSITY OF WISCONSIN—MADISON
Madison, Wisconsin

INSTITUTE FOR ENVIRONMENTAL STUDIES

The Institute for Environmental Studies offers opportunities for undergraduate and graduate students who, when they are graduated, will participate in professions which relate to the man-environment system.

Faculty associated with IES are currently preparing campus-wide Environmental Studies programs, including proposals for degrees on both the undergraduate and graduate (M.S., Ph.D.) levels. The planning includes:

(1) A broad undergraduate program which will develop environmental management skills and which will contribute to a knowledgeable and ecologically perceptive citizenry.

(2) A master's level program for training environmental managers.

(3) Master's and doctoral research programs directed particularly at interdisciplinary environmental areas, including environmental modeling, which are not now developed in discipline-oriented programs.

(4) An adult education and extension program to carry the results of University research to application on the many pressing environmental problems, and to provide an interchange of ideas between the university and citizens.

Degrees in Environmental Studies, per se, are not available at the University of Wisconsin—Madison at this time. However, students may get involved in this area through association with IES, a number of cross-departmental programs, and a wide variety of departments currently emphasizing environmental studies.

For further information, contact:

Professor Reid A. Bryson, Director
Institute for Environmental Studies
The University of Wisconsin—Madison
1225 West Dayton Street
Madison, Wisconsin 53706

WORCHESTER POLYTECHNIC INSTITUTE
Worchester, Massachusetts

ENVIRONMENTAL SYSTEMS STUDY

The Environmental Systems Study Program at WPI is an experimental program to develop an Interdisciplinary Project Approach in Education. The ESSP, established through a grant from the Alfred P. Sloan Foundation and coordinating with cooperating Industrial and Governmental agencies, will emphasize air, water, and solid waste environmental problems.

This is not a degree program. The student remains in his chosen department and may be allowed to use electives or to adjust his departmental schedule in order to elect the environmental, interdisciplinary or systems design course work related to the problem.

The student, under the guidance of a faculty advisor, will:

(1) Participate on an interdisciplinary team;
(2) Work on a real engineering problem;
(3) Develop knowledge of the Environment;
(4) Contribute to the improvement of the Environment; and
(5) Gain experience for future employment.

For more information, contact:

Mr. Joseph Mielinski, Administrator
Environmental Systems Study Office
Salisbury 04
Worchester Polytechnic Institute
Worchester, Massachusetts 01609

The following schools offer the undergraduate a considerable number of courses in the Environmental Sciences.

Adrian College
Adrian, Michigan 49221

Alaska Methodist University
Anchorage, Alaska 99504

Alliance College
Cambridge Springs, Pa. 16403

Andrews University
Berrien Springs, Mich. 49104

Butler University
Indianapolis, Indiana 46208

The Catholic University of
America
Washington, DC 20017

Central Missouri State
College
Warrensburg, Missouri 64093

Coe College
Cedar Rapids, Iowa 52402

The Colorado College
Colorado Springs, Colo. 80903

Concordia College
Physics Department
Moorhead, Minnesota 56560

Fairfield University
Fairfield, Connecticut 06430

Grinnel College
Grinnel, Iowa 50122

University of Hartford
200 Bloomfield Avenue
West Hartford, Conn. 06117

Kent State University
Kent, Ohio 44242

Kirkland College
Clinton, New York 13323

Know College
Galesburg, Illinois 61401

Lamar University
Beaumont, Texas 77705

Loma Linda University
Loma Linda, California 92354

Louisiana State University in
New Orleans
Lake Front
New Orleans, Louisiana 70122

Louisiana Tech University
Ruston, Louisiana 71270

Lowell Technological
Institute
Lowell, Massachusetts 01854

Malone College
Canton, Ohio 44709

Marlboro College
Marlboro, Vermont 05344

Mercy College of Detroit
8200 W. Outer Drive
Detroit, Michigan 48219

Messiah College
Grantham, Penna. 17027

Mississipi State College for
Women
Columbus, Mississippi 39701

The U. of North Carolina at
Asheville
Asheville, N.C. 28801

University of Northern
Colorado
Greeley, Colorado 80631
(This school has minor fields
of study in the
Environmental Sciences.)

Northern Illinois State
College
Bryn Mawr at St. Louis Ave.
Chicago, Illinois 60625

Northern Illinois University
Dekalb, Illinois 60115

Oakland University
Rochester, Michigan 48063

Old Dominion University
Norfolk, Virginia 23508

The Philadelphia College of
Pharmacy & Science
43 Street, Kingsessing &
Woodland Avenues
Philadelphia, Penna. 19104

Portland State University
Porland, Oregon 97207

Radford College
Radford, Virginia 24141

St. John Fisher College
Rochester, New York 14618

Saint Mary of the Plains
College
Dodge City, Kansas 67801

San Fernando Valley State
College
Northridge, California 91324

Sarah Lawrence College
Bronxville, New York 10708
(Freshman studies in the
Environmental Sciences)

Seattle Pacific College
Seattle, Washington 98119

University of South Carolina
Columbia, S.C. 29208

Southwestern At Memphis
2000 North Parkway
Memphis, Tennessee 38112

Stanislaus State College
800 Monte Vista Avenue
Turlock, California 95380

State University College at
Oneonta
Oneonta, New York 13820

The State University College
at Potsdam
Potsdam, New York 13676

The State University of
New York at Oswego
Oswego, New York 13126

Temple Buell College
1800 Pontiac Street
Denver, Colorado 80220

Transylvania University
Lexington, Kentucky 40508

Villanova University
Villanova, Pennsylvania 19085

Wartburg College
Waverly, Iowa 50677

Washington and Jefferson
College
Washington, Penna. 15301

Weber State College
Ogden, Utah 84403

Wesleyan University
Middletown, Conn. 06457

West Virginia Institute of
Technology
Montgomery, W.Va. 25136

Westmont College
Santa Barbara, Calif. 93103

Wheaton College
Wheaton, Illinois 60187

Wisconsin State University
Superior, Wisconsin 54881

The following schools have proposed programs for undergraduate degrees in Environmental Science. In most cases these programs are close to becoming part of the school's degree offerings.

Bowdoin College
Brunswick, Maine 04011

Florida Institute of
   Technology
Melbourne, Florida 32901

Fresno State College
Fresno, California 93710

Hunter College
790 Madison Avenue
New York, N.Y. 10021
(Hunter College has a 60
   credit Masters Program in
   Urban Planning)

Lake Erie College
Painesville, Ohio 44077

University of Nevada
Reno, Nevada 89507

Nichols College
Dudley, Massachusetts 01570

Northeastern University
Boston, Massachusetts 02115

Oregon State University
Corvallis, Oregon 97331

Southwestern College
Winfield, Kansas 67156

Ursinus College
Collegeville, Penna. 19426

Utah State University
Logan, Utah 84321

STUDENT ENVIRONMENTAL PROJECTS . . .

In December 1971, some 500 students from 97 colleges and universities met in Philadelphia, Pa., to present a series of papers on environmental problems as part of the 138th annual meeting of the American Association for the Advancement of Science. The topics varied over a wide range of subjects; some students, using standard scientific methods, proved hypotheses about the earth's processes; others found that their ideas were false. And learned by that finding, also.

When a group of San Jose State College students got together last year to study environmental health and the quality of life, for example, they speculated that three things would be true: that attitudes toward urban environment would vary in relation to home and neighborhood environment; that physical health would vary in relation to home and neighborhood environment; and that the quality of home and neighborhood environment would vary with the priority placed by city government on environmental considerations.

They found that they were two-thirds wrong.

The group revealed that the commonly held attitudes toward the environment and those active in protecting it are, for the most part, erroneous.

Instead of verifying their original assumptions, the researchers found that:

"(1) Those affected the most by environmental deterioration are more sensitive to it than those least affected. This finding is inconsistent with popular belief, which identifies environmental concerns with higher socio-economic status, and this finding requires a refinement in distinctions about who is concerned with what in the environmental movement today.

"(2) Those affected the most by environmental deterioration are less likely to exercise their right to vote than those least affected. This behavior is commonly associated with the feeling of discontent for the present means to bring about institutional change, specifically change required to 'better their environmental lot.'

"(3) Neighborhood environmental conditions are not solely attributable to the impact of the local residents. Forces beyond the control of local residents most certainly have major effects upon local conditions. Environmental quality is directly affected by a city's planning decisions; and the absence of a strict regulatory policy and direction is as detrimental to a city's quality of life as several loosely enforced, growth-related policies.

"(4) Factors related to personal histories and current life styles have stronger effects on environmental attitudes and behavior than a neighborhood's physical environment. Or alternatively, it may be concluded that levels of pollution concentrations, population densities and information gathered by [the group's testing methods] do not adequately define the immediate physical environment."

Although the work, as the report notes, "posed more questions than it provided answers," the researchers point out one important finding: "The failure of this study to support clearly all of the adopted hypotheses increases one's awareness of the complexity of relations among demographic factors, attitudes, urban planning and environmental quality, and cautions one against drawing premature conclusions."

The report also condemns the San Jose city government and people for their lack of foresight, noting:

"One would have to be a dreamer to suggest that San Jose could have remained an agriculturally-based community. That a change would occur was, and is, undeniable. But San Jose could have become something far greater than the model of urban sprawl it is today. Given a far-sighted government and a more civic-minded populace, it could have become an urban center in a natural setting, much as Monte Sereno and Saratoga, two other Santa Clara County communities, did during the late 1950s. That it did not is an almost tragic reminder that governments do not always make the best decisions possible."

The following list contains the names of the student project directors who presented the reports at the AAAS meeting and the titles of their research projects.

Their schools undoubtedly had the facilities they needed to perform their research. And if the topics of some of the papers below interest you, we suggest you write to their authors and find out just what their school has to offer. The best advice can come from someone who has been there.

Mr. Andrew C. Rucks
c/o Dr. Hal B. Pickle
School of Business
Auburn University
Auburn, Ala. 36830

Air and Water Pollution Control by the Textile Industry in the Southeast

Mr. Bryan MacLean
c/o Dr. Robert B. Weeden
Department of Wildlife Management
University of Alaska
College, Alaska 99701

Resource Utilization and Environmental Contamination in a Rapidly Changing Alaskan Eskimo Village

Mr. Garry R. Allen
c/o Dr. William Gensler
Department of Electrical Engineering
University of Arizona
Tucson, Ariz. 85721

Atmospheric Dispersion of Sulfur Dioxide from Copper Smelters

Mr. John H. Robinson
c/o Mr. S. Ernest Swickard
School of Architecture
California State Polytechnic College
San Luis Obispo, Calif. 93401

Socio-Economic Impact of the Palmdale Intercontinental Airport on a Desert Region of Los Angeles County

Mr. Philip J. Riggan
c/o Dr. Paul H. Zedler
Deparment of Biology
San Diego State College
San Diego, Calif. 92115

Physical, Biological, and Sociological Effects of Chaparral Fires in Southern California

Mr. Mark Tigan
c/o Dr. Donald W. Aitken
Department of Environmental Studies
San Jose State College
San Jose, Calif. 95114

Relationship of Environmental Quality to Human Health and the "Quality of life"

Miss Sharron L. Mee
c/o Dr. James B. Gale
Department of Physical Education
Sonoma State College
Rohnert Park, Calif. 94928

Physiological Effects of Exercising in a Polluted Atmosphere

Mr. Charles W. Horton c/o Dr. J. Richard Phillips Department of Engineering Harvey Mudd College Claremont, Calif. 91711	Mathematical Models and Computer Simulation of Smog Production in the Pomona Valley of California
Mr. Mark R. Shelley c/o Dr. Welton L. Lee Department of Biology Stanford University Stanford, Calif. 94305	Effects of Sewage Discharge on Monterey Bay
Miss Lynne Diane Houck c/o Dr. Patrick J. Pagni Department of Mechanical Engineering University of California Berkeley, Calif. 94720	Forest Fire Research: Control, Data Acquisition, and Modeling
Mr. Robert Dale Kelso c/o Dr. Herbert G. Baker Department of Botany University of California Berkeley, Calif. 94720	Grazing Pressure and Successional Changes in the Biotic Communities of the Point Reyes National Seashore
Mr. Richard W. Carey c/o Dr. Robert W. Gill Department of Life Sciences University of California Riverside, Calif. 92502	Development of Environmental Curriculum Resource Materials for Grades 4 through 12
Mr. James R. Zuboy c/o Dr. Howard Alden Department of Outdoor Recreation Colorado State University Fort Collins, Colo. 80521	Development of a Multiple Use Plan for the Colorado State Forest
Mr. Eloy Soza c/o Dr. Ralph E. Williams Department of Mechanical Sciences and Environmental Engineering University of Denver Denver, Colo. 80210	Design of a Migrant and Rural Farm Worker Housing Community
Mr. Glenn R. Harris c/o Dr. Jelle de Boer Department of Geology Wesleyan University Middletown, Conn. 06457	Feasibility Study of Quarries as Dumping Sites for Disposal of Solid Wastes
Mr. Mark Graustein c/o Dr. Norman F. Collins Department of Agricultural Engineering University of Delaware Newark, Del. 19711	The Role of Insects in Animal and Processing Plant Waste Breakdown
Mr. Kenneth Strom c/o Dr. Leopold May Department of Chemistry The Catholic University of America Washington, D.C. 20017	Some Ecological Effects of Sanitary Landfills
Mr. Sam S. Hill, III c/o Dr. J. Richard Warren Director, Continuing Education Jacksonville University Jacksonville, Fla. 32211	Design of an Urban Transportation System for Jacksonville, Florida
Mr. Paul Carlson c/o Dr. John B. Morrill Chairman, Department of Natural Sciences New College Sarasota, Fla. 33578	Ecological Effects of Spoil Islands Created by Dredging in Estuaries along the West Coast of Florida

Mr. Peter M. Hahn
c/o Dr. M. W. Anderson
Department of Structures,
  Materials, Fluids
University of South Florida
Tampa, Fla. 33620

Characteristics, Potential Uses, and
Control of the Water Hyacinth

Mr. Patrick H. Neale
c/o Dr. Carl H. Snyder
Department of Chemistry
University of Miami
Coral Gables, Fla. 33124

Chemical and Biological Relationships
in Deep Water Areas of the
Everglades

Mr. Jerrold Hornstein
School of Industrial and
  Systems Engineering
Georgia Institute of Technology
Atlanta, Ga. 30332

Relationships between the Proposed
Rapid Transit System, the
Environment, and Sociological Factors
in Atlanta

Mr. Steven L. Montgomery
c/o Dr. D. Elmo Hardy
Department of Entomology
University of Hawaii
Honolulu, Hawaii 96822

Ecology of the Hawaiian Drylands

Mr. Michael Osato
c/o Dr. John G. Chan
University of Hawaii, Hilo College
Hilo, Hawaii 96720

Biological, Chemical, and Sociological
Consequences of Pollution in
Hilo Bay, Hawaii

Mr. David Maxfield
c/o Dr. Chien M. Wai
Department of Chemistry
University of Idaho
Moscow, Idaho 83843

Heavy Metal Pollution in Sediments
of the Coeur d'Alene River Delta

Mr. Richard C. Stupka
c/o Dr. James E. Brower
Department of Biological Sciences
Northern Illinois University
DeKalb, Ill. 60115

Lead Pollution Effects on Terrestrial
and Aquatic Ecosystems of the
Great Lakes Region

Mr. Daniel L. Eberhardt
c/o Dr. Claude A. Lucchesi
Director of Analytical Services
Northwestern University
Evanston, Ill. 60201

Chemical, Biological, and Economic
Studies of Muncipal Garbage
Composting

Miss Christine Lehto
c/o Dr. Sol Tax
Department of Anthropology
University of Chicago
Chicago, Ill. 60637

Migration of Rural Indians to
Urban Centers

Mr. Richard C. Frederick or
Mr. Dale R. Jurich
c/o Dr. William Randolph Boggess
Department of Forestry
University of Illinois
Urbana, Ill. 61801

Effects on Society and the
Environment of Alternative Methods
of Packaging Goods for Household
Consumption

Mr. Hector J. Rosquete
c/o Dr. John E. Christian
Institute for Environmental Health
Purdue University
Lafayette, Ind. 47907

Air Pollution, Water Pollution, and
Solid Waste Disposal Problems in
the Greater Lafayette Area, Indiana

Mr. Anthony J. Wheeler
c/o Dr. Kenneth A. Christiansen
Department of Biology
Grinnell College
Grinnell, Iowa 50112

Biological and Chemical Levels of
Pollution in Rock Creek Lake, Iowa

Mr. Edwin J. Spicka
c/o Dr. Ronald W. Turner
Department of Biology
St. Benedict's College
Atchison, Kan. 66002

Air and Water Pollution in the
Atchison, Kansas, Area

Mr. Douglas K. Nelson
c/o Dr. Walter Bernhart
Department of Aeronautical
  Engineering
Wichita State University
Wichita, Kan. 67208

Determination of Levels and
Distribution of Noise in Wichita,
Kansas

Mr. Gary Harlow
c/o Dr. Donald Rowe
Department of Engineering
  Technology
Western Kentucky University
Bowling Green, Ky. 42101

Water Quality of Barren River,
Kentucky

Mr. Welton C. Washington
c/o Dr. Franklin D. Hill
Department of Chemistry
Grambling College
Grambling, La. 71245

Blood Levels of DDT as a Function
of Race, Habitat, and Socio-economic
Status

Mr. Michael R. Howard
c/o Dr. John W. Rock
Department of Architecture
Tulane University
New Orleans, La. 70118

Links between Life Style and
Environmental Expression in
Building, Past and Present

Mr. Richard Alan Cohen
c/o Dr. Dana W. Mayo
Department of Chemistry
Bowdoin College
Brunswick, Maine 04011

Detection and Estimation of Natural
Regeneration Processes in the Upper
Androscoggin River, Maine

Mr. Joseph M. Wunderle, Jr.
c/o Dr. Ronald B. Davis
Department of Botany and Geology
University of Maine at Orono
Orono, Maine 04473
*Physical, Ecological, Economic and
Sociological Effects of Residence Patterns
of Recreationists on Four Maine Lakes*

Mr. Bruce Pollock Thompson
c/o Dr. Stuart Fisher
Department of Biology
Amherst College
Amherst, Mass. 01002
*Quantification of the Relationships
between Land Use and Water Quality
in the Fort River, Massachusetts*

Miss Virginia L. Richards
c/o Dr. John W. Foerster
Department of Biological Science
Goucher College
Towson, Md. 21204
*Analysis of Degradation of Lake Roland,
Baltimore*

Mr. Stephen P. Gormican
c/o Reverend James W. Skehan, S.J.
Director, Environmental Center
Boston College
Chestnut Hill, Mass. 02167
*Scientific, Legal, Sociological and
Psychological aspects of Pollution of
Lake Cochituate, Massachusetts*

Mr. Gary C. Stanton
c/o Dr. Zigfridas Vaituzis
Department of Microbiology
University of Maryland
College Park, Md. 20742
*Extent and Sources of Pollution in
Rock Creek, Maryland and the District
of Columbia*

Mr. Earl Strayhorn
c/o Dr. J. C. Edozien
Department of Nutrition & Food
  Science
Massachusetts Institute of Technology
Cambridge, Mass. 02139
*Nutrition as Related to General Health
Status of a Segment of the Greater
Boston Community*

Mr. Noah Bass
c/o Dr. Rainer A. Weiss
Department of Physics
Massachusetts Institute of Technology
Cambridge, Mass. 02139
*Atmospheric Pollution Due to Gases of
Simple Molecular Structure*

Mr. John Thomas
c/o Dr. Ronald A. Parejko
Department of Biology
Northern Michigan University
Marquette, Mich. 49855
*Feasibility of Producing and Marketing a
Soil-Like Product from Municipal Wastes
and Mine Tailings*

Mr. Roger D. Brooks
c/o Dr. Keith R. Kleckner
Department of Engineering
Oakland University
Rochester, Mich. 48063
*Power Train Design for an Electrically-
Powered Automobile*

Miss Barbara J. Pickens
c/o Dr. John Loss
School of Architecture
University of Detroit
Detroit, Mich. 48221
*Relationship between Changes in Physical
Dwelling Unit Environment and
Social Environment*

Miss Suzanne C. Pick
c/o Dr. Howard Schuman
Department of Sociology
University of Michigan
Ann Arbor, Mich. 48104
*Attitudes of Working Mothers toward
Child Care Centers*

Mr. Sander H. Orent
c/o Dr. Steven Hubbell
Department of Zoology
University of Michigan
Ann Arbor, Mich. 48104
*Biological and Economic Aspects of
Predator (Coyote) Control*

Mr. Michael R. Cunningham
c/o Dr. Arthur L. Buikema, Jr.
Department of Biology
St. Olaf College
Northfield, Minn. 55057
Carleton College
Northfield, Minn. 55057
*Behavior and Attitudes of Vacationers in
Wilderness Areas of Superior National
Forest and Boundary Waters Canoe
Area, Minnesota*

Mr. Gregg Shadduck
c/o Dr. Alan H. Humphreys
Department of Elementary Education
University of Minnesota
Minneapolis, Minn. 55455
*Development of Environmental Studies
Blocks for High School Students*

Mr. Burke West
c/o Dr. John W. Legg
Department of Chemistry
Mississippi College
Clinton, Miss. 39056
*Lead and Gaseous Pollutants along
Newly-Built and Old Highways*

Mr. David Slusher
c/o Dr. Stanley E. Manahan
Department of Chemistry
University of Missouri
Columbia, Mo. 65201
*Possible Heavy Metal Ion Transport by
Trisodium Nitriloacetate (NTA) in Waste
Treatment Plants and Aquatic Ecosystems*

Mr. Mark Young
c/o Dr. P. J. Reilly
Department of Chemical Engineering
University of Nebraska
Lincoln, Neb. 68508
*Preparation of Salable By-Products
through Aerobic Fermentation of
Paunch Liquors*

Mr. Jeffrey W. Bock
c/o Dr. Charles L. Braun
Department of Chemistry
Dartmouth College
Hanover, N.H. 03755
*A study of Biological, Chemical, and
Sociological Aspects of Pollution of
Mascoma Lake, New Hampshire*

Mr. James A. Philbrook
c/o Dr. William A. Hunzeker
Department of Management
    Information Systems
New Hampshire College
Manchester, N.H. 03101
*Evaluation of Project Head Start in Con-
trasting Urban and Rural Areas of
New Hampshire*

Mr. Thomas J. Givnish
c/o Dr. David J. J. Kinsman
Department of Geology &
    Geophysical Sciences
Princeton University
Princeton, N.J. 08504
*Impact of Proposed Watershed Changes
on Ecology of New Jersey Pine Barrens*

Mr. John Gragg
c/o Dr. Roshan B. Bhappu
Department of Metallurgy
New Mexico Institute of Mining
    and Technology
Socorro, N.M. 87801
*Survey of Water Quality, Soils, and Crops
along the Irrigation Canal near Socorro,
New Mexico*

Mr. Joseph E. Schwartz
c/o Dr. L. Reissman
Department of Sociology
Cornell University
Ithaca, N.Y. 14850
*Appropriateness of Current Designs of
Low Income Housing*

Miss Gloria Gardocki
c/o Dr. Philip H. Ramsey
Department of Psychology
Hofstra University
Hempstead, N.Y. 11550
The Social, Psychological, and
Demographic Variables which Influence
Family Size and Population Growth Rates

Mr. George Panoussis
c/o Dr. P. C. Wang
Department of Civil Engineering
Polytechnic Institute of Brooklyn
Brooklyn, N.Y. 11201
Engineering and Psychological Studies of
Vibrations in New York

Mr. Walter K. Muench
c/o Dr. J. L. McHugh
Department of Marine Resources
State University of New York-
  Stony Brook
Stony Brook, N.Y. 11790
An Environmental Study of Long Island's
Mount Sinai Harbor

Mr. Robert Bannister
c/o Dr. Harold Kibby
Department of Biological Sciences
State University of New York-
  Brockport
Brockport, N.Y. 14420
Pollution Survey of the New York State
Barge Canal

Mr. Paul Feldsher or
Miss Susan B. Williams
c/o Dr. William P. Mangin
Department of Anthropology
Syracuse University
Syracuse, N.Y. 13210
Sociological Impact of Radical
Environmental Change on a Group of
Seneca Indians

Mr. Gregory Keating Hearn
c/o Dr. Edward M. Brody
Institute of Optics
University of Rochester
Rochester, N.Y. 14627
Use of Light Scattering Techniques to
Detect and Measure Particulate Matter
in Water

Mr. Stephen B. Benton
c/o Mr. C. W. O'Rear
Department of Biology
East Carolina University
Greenville, N.C. 27834
Pollution Studies of the Tar River
Tributaries in North Carolina

Miss Karen Cummings
c/o Dr. Fred Holtkamp
Department of Chemistry
Mars Hill College
Mars Hill, N.C. 28754
Local Conditions and Practices
Contributing to Environmental
Degradation in a Rural Appalachian
County in North Carolina

Mr. Thomas P. Graham
c/o Dr. John C. Bernhard, Jr.
Department of Biology
University of North Carolina—
  Asheville
Asheville, N.C. 28801
Ecological Effects of Hot Water
Discharged by an Electric Power
Generating Plant

Mrs. Adelaide Anne Williams
c/o Dr. Peter D. Weigl
Department of Biology
Wake Forest University
Winston-Salem, N.C. 27109
Residue Levels of Chlorinated
Hydrocarbons in Mammals as a Function
of Geographic Region and Land Use in
North Carolina

Mr. Gregory L. Olson
c/o Dr. Robert D. Koob
Department of Chemistry
North Dakota State University
Fargo, N.D. 58102
Study of Air Water Pollutants and their
Relationships

Mr. Steven Bill
c/o Dr. Robert G. Rolan
Department of Biology
Cleveland State University
Cleveland, Ohio 44115
History of Eutrophication Cycles in Lake
Erie Derived from Bottom Core Samples

Mr. W. Gregory Lotz
c/o Dr. Martin Reno
Department of Physics
Heidelberg College
Tiffin, Ohio 44883
Pollution in the Sandusky River, Ohio

Mr. John Barone
c/o Dr. G. Dennis Cooke
Department of Biological Sciences
Kent State University
Kent, Ohio 44240
Heavy Metal Pollutants in a Section of
the Cuyahoga River Watershed

Mr. Harvey P. Cahoon
c/o Dr. Ivan B. Cutler
Department of Material Science &
  Engineering
University of Utah
Salt Lake City, Utah 84112
Feasibility of Making Insulation Material
by Foaming Waste Glass

Mr. Gregory S. Trutza
c/o Dr. John D. Briggs
College of Biological Sciences
Ohio State University
Columbus, Ohio 43210
Biological Controls for Protecting Sweet
Corn from the Corn Earworm

Mr. Mark MacNealy
c/o Dr. Joseph D. Laufersweiler
Department of Biology
University of Dayton
Dayton, Ohio 45409
Control of Ozone and Titanium Dioxide
Pollution by the Use of Antioxidants

Mr. W. Lawrence Harvey
c/o Dr. Louis H. Summers
Department of Architecture and
  Civil Engineering
University of Oklahoma
Norman, Okla. 73069
*The Effect of Urban Change on "The
Square" of Courthouse Square Towns*

Mr. J. Peterson Myers
c/o Dr. Jeffrey Kelly
Department of Chemistry
Reed College
Portland, Ore. 97202
*Political, Sociological, Economic, and
Biological Considerations Affecting a
Predator Control Program in the Steens
Mountains of Eastern Oregon*

Mr. Edward McConnaughey
c/o Dr. Paul Rudy
Director-Institute of Marine Biology
University of Oregon
Eugene, Ore. 97403
*An Integrated Land and Water Use Plan
for the Coos Bay Estuary*

Mr. Lawrence J. Young
c/o Dr. John C. Purcupile
Department of Mechanical
  Engineering
Carnegie-Mellon University
Pittsburgh, Pa. 15213
*Production of Protein by Single-Celled
Organisms Grown in Municipal
Liquid Wastes*

Mr. Richard Blutstein
c/o Dr. Robert E. Leyon
Department of Chemistry
Dickinson College
Carlisle, Pa. 17013
*Effects of Municipal, Residential, and
Industrial Sewage and Solid Wastes on
Two Tributaries of the Susquehanna River*

Mr. Gary W. Jay
c/o Dr. Kenneth H. Brookshire
Department of Psychology
Franklin and Marshall College
Lancaster, Pa. 17604
*Effects of Mercury Compounds on the
Central Nervous Systems of Fish*

Mr. Vaughn L. Glasgow
c/o Dr. W. R. Weisman
Department of Art History
Pennsylvania State University
University Park, Pa. 16802
*A Socio-Historic Determination of Cast
Iron Structures in the So-Ho District of
New York City*

Mr. Marlin L. Hornberger
c/o Dr. Edwin L. Cooper
Department of Biology
Pennsylvania State University
University Park, Pa. 16802
*Biological and Chemical Effects of Land
Use on Little Pine Creek, Pennsylvania*

Mr. Keith G. Kirk
c/o Dr. A. L. Guber
College of Earth and Mineral Sciences
Pennsylvania State University
University Park, Pa. 16802
*The Effectiveness of Backfilling in
Controlling Acid Mine Drainage in the
Allegheny Plateau of Pennsylvania*

Mr. John H. Flaschen
c/o Dr. John Imbrie
Department of Geological Sciences
Brown University
Providence, R.I. 02912
*Water Quality Problems in the Pawtuxent
River Basin, Rhode Island*

Mr. James E. McCoy
c/o Dr. David E. Shulenburger
Department of Economics
Clemson University
Clemson, S.C. 29631
*Physical Mobility of the Aged in a
Southern City and its Effects on their
Socio-Economic Environment*

Mr. Jesse Wolf
c/o Sister Kieran Diggins
Department of Biology
Mount Marty College
Yankton, S.D. 57078
*Benthic Organisms in Natural and
Channelized Portions of the Missouri River*

Mr. Douglas S. Shafer
c/o Dr. Joe A. Chapman
Department of Biology
Carson-Newman College
Jefferson City, Tenn. 37760
*Level of Pollutants and Bacteria in the
Underground Waters of East Tennessee*

Mr. Allen Warner Phelps
c/o Dr. Bobby R. Jones
Department of Biology
Southwestern at Memphis
Memphis, Tenn. 38112
*Pathways by Which Mercury is
Introduced into an Ecosystem*

Mr. Donald Robert Quartel, Jr.
c/o Dr. Brien Ralph Hammond
Department of Biology
William Marsh Rice University
Houston, Tex. 77001
*Mercury Concentrations in Gulf Coast
Mullet and the Mullet Food Chain*

Mr. Alex F. Sears
c/o Dr. George O. Elle
Department of Agronomy
Texas Tech University
Lubbock, Tex. 79409
*Quality of Source Water for Proposed
Recreational Lakes in Yellowstone Canyon
near Lubbock, Texas*

Department of Biology
University of Utah
Salt Lake City, Utah 84112
*Ecology of Antelope Island and
Farmington Bay Area of Great Salt Lake*

Mr. Richard H. Fuller
c/o Dr. Raymond L. Kerns, Jr.
Department of Geology
Utah State University
Logan, Utah 84321
*The Extent of Pollution and its Control
in the Bear Lake Basin*

Mr. Wayne Timura
c/o Dr. William J. Jewell
Department of Civil Engineering
University of Vermont
Burlington, Vt. 05401
*Analysis of Transportation and
Environmental Resources of the
Waterfront in Burlington, Vermont*

Mr. John F. Batkins
c/o Dr. Robert L. Ake
Department of Chemistry
Old Dominion University
Norfolk, Va. 23508
Land Use Planning in Virginia Beach

Miss Anne H. Lindsey
c/o Dr. Franklin F. Flint
Department of Biology
Randolph-Macon Woman's College
Lynchburg, Va. 24504
*Ecological Study of Blackwater Creek
Basin, Preliminary to its Development as
a Park in Lynchburg, Virginia*

Mr. John G. Comis
c/o Dr. E. B. Welch
Department of Civil Engineering
Water and Air Resources
University of Washington
Seattle, Wash. 98105
*Water Quality Study of Swamp and
Coal Creeks, King County, Washington*

Department of Theoretical and
Applied Mechanics
West Virginia University
Morgantown, W. Va. 26506
Noise Abatement in Dormitories

Mr. David Radloff
c/o Dr. Richard E. Bayer
Department of Chemistry
Carroll College
Waukesha, Wis. 53186
*Measurement and Control of Feed Lot
Pollution*

Mr. Jacob J. Emmerick
c/o Dr. Robert E. Bowman
Department of Psychology
University of Wisconsin
Madison, Wis. 53706
*Effects of Overcrowding on the Behavior
and Biochemistry of Primate Groups*

Mr. Paul Lewis
c/o Dr. Dennis H. Knight
Department of Botany
University of Wyoming
Laramie, Wyo. 82070
*Commercial Clear-Cutting in High
Altitude Forests of Wyoming*

. . . AND OTHER SOURCES

The people listed below may be contacted for more information concerning their research in the environmental field and the schools with which they are associated. Their fields are specialized; but, perhaps, so are your interests.

Municipal and Solid Waste Management

Prof. Percy H. McGauhey
Sanitary Engineering Research
Laboratory
University of California
Richmond Field Station
Berkeley, California 94804
*Research program on solid waste
management*

Dr. Clarence Golueke
University of California
Sanitary Engineering Research
Laboratory
1301 S. 46 Street
Richmond, California 94804
Member, Compost Science Editorial Board

Howard L. Selznick
Department of Civil Engineering
Stanford University
Stanford, California 94305

Seymour S. Block
Department Chemical Engineering
University of Florida
Gainesville, Florida

Thomas DeS. Furman
Prof. Environmental Engr.
Envir. Engr. Dept.
University of Florida
Gainesville, Florida 32601

Dr. Frederick G. Pohland
School of Civil Engineering
Georgia Institute Technology
Atlanta, Georgia 30332

Dr. B. C. Spradlin
School Industrial Engineering
Georgia Institute of Technology
Atlanta, Georgia

Dr. Fred C. Gurnham
Illinois Institute Technology
3200 S. Wabash Avenue
IIT Center
Chicago, Illinois 60616
Research on handling solid wastes

Dr. John R. Sheaffer
Center Urban Studies
University of Chicago
Chicago, Illinois 60601

Wesley D. Bonds, Jr.
Northwestern University
Evanson, Illinois 60201

Dr. Ross E. McKinney
Chairman, Dept. Civil Engineering
University of Kansas
Lawrence, Kansas
Pollution-free disposal techniques

Kazi F. Jalal
Harvard University
Cambridge, Massachusetts
*A Technological Evaluation of
Composting for Community Waste
Disposal in Asia*

Dr. David G. Wilson
Dept. Mechanical Engineering
M.I.T.
Cambridge, Massachusetts
Member, Compost Science Editorial Board

Prof. Marshall I. Goldman
Wellesley College
Department of Economics
Wellesley, Massachusetts 02181

Lloyd L. Kempe
Prof. Chem. Eng. Microbiol.
University of Michigan
Ann Arbor, Michigan 48104

William Stapp
University of Michigan
Ann Arbor, Michigan

K. L. Schulze, Associate Prof.
Division of Engineering Research
Michigan State University
Lansing, Michigan
Member, Compost Science Editorial Board

Dr. Lloyd R. Robinson
Mississipi State University
Department Civil Engineering
P.O. Box 1321
State College, Mississippi 39762

Robert E. Kohn
Washington University
St. Louis, Missouri
The Economics of Using Leaves

Raul R. Cardenas, Jr.
New York University
Civil Engineering Department
Bronx, New York 20453

Walter R. Lynn, Director
Center for Environmental Quality
 Management
Cornell University
302 Hollister Hall
Ithaca, New York 14850

Nicholas L. Clesceri, Ph.D.
Environmental Engineering
Rensselaer Polytechnic Institute
Troy, New York 12181

William S. Galler
Associate Prof. Civil Engineering
North Carolina State University
Raleigh, North Carolina
*Physical and Chemical Analysis of
Domestic Municipal Refuse From Raleigh*

Lawrence J. Partridge, Jr.
North Carolina State University
Raleigh, North Carolina
*Physical and Chemical Analysis of
Domestic Municipal Refuse from Raleigh*

Dr. A. A. Fungaroli
Drexel University
32 & Chestnut Streets
Philadelphia, Pennsylvania 19104

Dr. Ruth Patrick
Chairman Department of Limnology
Academy of Natl. Sciences of Phila.
Philadelphia, Pennsylvania

Prof. John B. Nesbitt
Pennsylvania State University
216 Sackett Bldg.
University Park, Pennsylvania 16801

Prof. Iraj Zandi
The Towne School of Civil &
 Mechanical Engineering
University of Pennsylvania
University Park, Pennsylvania
*Member, Compost Science Editorial
Board Pipeline Transport of Wastes*

Dr. Jean Gottman
Department of Geography
University of Wisconsin
Madison, Wisconsin

Robert K. Ham
Assistant Prof. Civil Engineering
3232 Eng. Bldg.
University of Wisconsin
Madison, Wisconsin 53706
Shredded Refuse

G. K. Voigt
University of Wisconsin
Madison, Wisconsin

Vinton W. Bacon
Civil Engineering
University of Wisconsin
Milwaukee, Wisconsin
Municipal Waste—Economics

Agriculture: Soil Application, Stabilization, Decomposition

Willis C. Martin, Jr.
Department of Horticulture
Auburn University
Mobile, Alabama

Henry P. Orr
Department of Horticulture
Auburn University
Mobile, Alabama

Kenneth C. Sanderson
Department of Horticulture
Auburn University
Mobile, Alabama

Professor D. G. Sturkie
Agronomy and Soils Dept.
Auburn University
Auburn, Alabama 36830

Dr. Wallace H. Fuller
Head of Department
Agricultural Chemistry & Soils
University of Arizona
Tucson, Arizona 85725
Compost & Soils Research

J. Vlamis
Dept. Soils & Plant Nutrition
University of California
Davis, Berkeley, California

Prof. W. J. Flocker
Dept. Agricultural Engineering
University of California
Davis, California 95616
Refuse Stabilization in the Land

Robert F. Heizer
Prof. Anthropology
University of California
Davis, California
Soil Organic Matter

G. K. York
Department of Food Science
University of California
Davis, California
Refuse Stabilization in the Land

G. J. Jann
Department of Bacteriology
University of California
Los Angeles, California

Prof. Charles Senn
University of California
Los Angeles, California
Composting manure

Dr. Cyrus M. McKell
Division of Agricultural Sciences
University of California
Riverside, California
Chicken manure

Dr. Charles C. Hortenstine
Dept. of Soils
University of Florida
Gainesville, Florida 32601
To determine effects of large amounts of compost on soil

Larry D. King
Department of Agronomy
University of Georgia
Athens, Georgia 30601

Silas McHenry
Associate Specialist in Poultry
  Husbandry
University of Hawaii, Honolulu
Poultry Manure Utilization

Dr. Roy E. Williams
Bureau of Mines and Geology
University of Idaho
Moscow, Idaho 83843
Waste water for irrigation

Dr. Donald L. Day
Dept. Agricultural Engineering
University of Illinois
Urbana, Illinois 61801
Develop methods of waste treatment/ management

J. W. Sicer
Poultry Science Department
Purdue University
Bloomington, Indiana
Poultry manure

Joe Berry, Assistant Professor
Purdue University
Poultry Building
W. Lafayette, Indiana 47907
Poultry Manure Management

E. Paul Taiganides
University of Iowa
Ames, Iowa
(Digestion of farm animal wastes)

D. L. Mader
U. of Massachusetts
Amherst, Massachusetts
Effect of humus on biocides in soil

Dr. William Albrecht
University of Missouri
Department of Soils
Columbia, Missouri 65201
Member, Compost Science Editorial Board

Harry E. Besley
Research Prof. Agricultural
  Engineering
Rutgers University
New Brunswick, New Jersey 08903
Agricultural Wastes

S. J. Toth
Professor of Soils
Rutgers University
New Brunswick, New Jersey
Member, Compost Science Editorial Board

E. E. Staffeldt
Assistant Professor Biology
New Mexico State University
Albuquerque, New Mexico

John S. Jeris
Civil Engineering Department
Manhattan College
Bronx, New York 10710
Decomposition of Cellulose and Refuse

Raymond W. Regan
Civil Engineering Department
Manhattan College
Bronx, New York 10710
Decomposition of Cellulose and Refuse

A. T. Sobel
Research Associate
Agricultural Engineering Department
Cornell University
Ithaca, New York
Block Drying of Chicken Manure

Prof. Albert Schatz
Temple University
Philadelphia, Pennsylvania 19119
Member, Compost Science Editorial Board

Herbert C. Jordan
Ag. Expt. Station
Pennsylvania State University
University Park, Pennsylvania
(Poultry Manure)

Zoell D. Colburn
Research Assistant
Ambassador College Agric.
  Department
Big Sandy, Texas 75755

D. J. Persidsky
University of Wisconsin
Madison, Wisconsin

Prof. Stanley A. Witzel
Agricultural Engineering
University of Wisconsin
Madison, Wisconsin 53706
*To evaluate economic value of farm
waste to agriculture*

Industrial Wastes

Dr. Charles F. Park, Jr.
Professor Geology & Mineral
  Engineering
Stanford University
Palo Alto, California

Dr. John Douros, Head
Microbiology Section, Chem. Div.
University of Denver
University Park
Denver, Colorado 80210
Degradation of waste paper to protein

Joel Giddens
Department of Agronomy
University of Georgia
Athens, Georgia
Cotton meal

Norman F. Oebker
Department of Horticulture
University of Illinois
Urbana, Illinois
Paper Mulch Studies

W. F. Echelberger, Jr.
University of Notre Dame
Notre Dame, Indiana
Fly-Ash Utilization

Mark W. Tenney
Associate Professor
Dept. of Engineering
University of Notre Dame
Notre Dame, Indiana
Fly-Ash Utilization

J. Clayton Herman
Cooperative Ext. Serv.
Iowa State University
Ames, Iowa 50010
Scrap collecting

Clayton D. Callihan
Dept. Chemical Engineering
Louisiana State University
Baton Rouge, Louisiana 70803
*The Economics of Microbial Proteins
Produced from Cellulosic Wastes*

Charles E. Dunlap
Dept. Chemical Eng.
Louisiana State University
Baton Rouge, Louisiana 70803
*The Economics of Microbial Proteins
Produced from Cellulosic Wastes*

Dr. Stuart Dunn
Plant Physiologist
University of New Hampshire
Durham, New Hampshire 03824
Wood Wastes

D. L. Downing
Department of Food Science &
  Technology
N. Y. Ag. Experiment Station
Cornell University
Geneva, New York 14456
*Problems with Processing Effluents in
the Food Industry*

D. F. Splittstoesser
Dept. Food Science & Technology
N. Y. Ag. Experiment Station
Cornell University
Geneva, New York 14456
*Problems with Processing Effluents in
the Food Industry*

Peter J. Barrer
Cornell Center Environmental Quality
Management
Ithaca, New York
Ecology and Junked Cars

Prof. Norman C. Dundero
Applied Microbiology
Cornell University
Ithaca, New York
Ecology & Junked Cars

B. G. Reeves
Ext. Cotton Gin Specialist
Texas A & M College
College Station, Texas

Prof. Stanley P. Gessel
Forest Soils
University of Washington
Seattle, Washington
Composted wood wastes

S. A Wilde
Professor of Soils
University of Wisconsin
Madison, Wisconsin

M. D. Woerpel
Wisconsin Alumni Research
    Foundation
University of Wisconsin
Madison, Wisconsin
Mechanization of the sawdust treatment

Sewage Sludge Utilization

Prof. A. D. Day
Arizona Ag. Expt. Stn.
Tucson, Arizona
(City Sewage Irrigation)

Richard Leslie Conn
University of Illinois
Chicago, Illinois
Liquid Sludge as a Farm Fertilizer

Dr. Tom Heinsley
College of Agriculture
University of Illinois
Chicago, Illinois
Sewage Sludge Effect on Soil

William E. Sopper
Prof. of Forest Hydrology
School of Forest Resources
The Pennsylvania State University
University Park, Pennsylvania 16802
*Irrigation With Municipal Sewage
Effluent & Sludge*

Prof. Edward L. Thackston
Sanitary and Water Resources
Vanderbilt University
Nashville, Tennessee 37203
Researcher on sanitary & water resources

Prof. James B. Reeves
Texas Western College
El Paso, Texas
(Composting sludge w/sawdust)

C. J. Chapman
Soils Department
University of Wisconsin
Madison, Wisconsin
(City Sewage Irrigation)

Wildlife Conservation Courses

This roster, prepared by the Wildlife Society, includes those North American campuses that have indicated they have special curricula related to the fields of wildlife conservation and management. This list is assembled for public service purposes only. It may not be complete, and it is not to be interpreted as any type of accreditation or certification or endorsement by The Wildlife Society. The minimum course requirements believed essential to anyone graduating with a Bachelor's Degree in wildlife, as adopted in March 1971 by the Wildlife Society, are appended to this roster as a useful guide to prospective wildlife students.

The different approaches to a higher education are sometimes difficult to decipher. It is hoped this "key" to the coding system used will be helpful in identifying properly the campuses of interest to you.

B   = Bachelors
M   = Masters
D   = Doctors
WP   = Wildlife
        Professor
S   = Has student
        chapter of
        The Wild-
        life Society

1 = Institution grants a named degree in wildlife.

2 = Institution grants a wildlife major option with degree in: a = Agriculture; b = Animal Science; c = Biology; d = Ecology; e = Education; f = Field Biology; g = Forestry; h = Parks; i = Range; j = Zoology.

3 = Institution grants no degree in wildlife, but may have curriculum or courses in wildlife.

ACADIA, U. of,
Wolfville, Nova Scotia
WP, Dept. Biol. (B3cM2c)

ALASKA, U. of,
College 99701
Head, Dept. Wildl. Mgt.
(BM1,D2c)

ALBERTA, U. of,
Edmonton, Can.
Head, Dept. Zool. (BMD3j)

ARIZONA, U. of,
Tucson 85721
Head, Dept. Biol. Sci.
(BM1, D3c)S

ARIZONA St. U.,
Tempe 85281
WP, Dept. Zool. (B1,MD3j)S

ARKANSAS Polytech. C.,
Russellville 72801
Head, Fish & Wildl. (B1)

AUBURN U.,
Auburn, Ala. 36830
Head, Dept. Zool.-Ent.
(B1,MD2j)S

S. F. AUSTIN St. C.,
Nachogdoches, Tex. 75961
WP, Biol. Dept. (BM3j)

BR. COLUMBIA, U. of,
Vancouver 8, Can.
WP, Dept. Zool. (BMD2agj)

CALIF. St. Poly. C.,
San Luis Obispo 93401
WP, Biol. Sci. Dept.
(BM3cfj)

CALIFORNIA, U. of,
Berkeley 94720
WP, School For. & Cons.
(BMD2gj)

CALIFORNIA, U. of,
Davis 95616
Chm., Dept. Animal
Physiology (B1)

CARLETON U.,
Ottawa, Ont., Can. (MD2cj)

CLEMSON U.,
Clemson, S.C. 29631
Head, Dept. Entom. & Zool.
(B3c,M1,D3j)

COLORADO St. U.,
Ft. Collins 80521
Head, Dept. Fish & Wildl.
Biol. (BMD1)S

CONNECTICUT, U. of,
Storrs 06268
Wildl. Ecol. Prof., Plant Sci.
Dept. (BM2)

CORNELL U.,
Ithaca, N.Y. 14850
Head, Dept. Cons. (BMD1)

FLORIDA, U. of,
Gainesville 32601
WP, School For.
(BM2g,D3bj)S

FLORIDA ATLANTIC U.,
Boca Raton 33432
(B3c)

GEORGIA, U. of,
Athens 30601
WP, School For. Res.
(BMD2g)S

GUELPH, U. of,
Guelph, Ont., Can.
Chm., Dept. Zool. (MD2j)S

HUMBOLDT St. C.,
Arcata, Cal. 95521
Chm., Div. Natural Res.
(BM1)

IDAHO, U. of, Moscow 83843
WP, Wildl. & Range Sci.
(BMD2g)S

IDAHO St. U.,
Pocatello 83201
Chm., Dept. Biol. (B1)

ILLINOIS, U. of,
Urbana 61801
WP, Dept. Zool. (BMD3cj)

NORTH. ILL. U.,
DeKalb 60115
(B3c)S

SOUTH. ILL. U.,
Carbondale 62901
WP, Dept. Zool (BMD3j)

WEST. ILL. U.,
Macomb 61455
WP, Dept. Biol. Sci. (BM3j)S

IOWA St. U., Ames 50010
WP, Dept. Zool. & Ent.
(B1MD2j)

KANSAS St. U.,
Manhattan 66502
WP, Div. Biol. (BMD2c)S

EAST. KENTUCKY U.,
Richmond 40475
Chm., Biol. Dept. (B1)

N.E. LOUISIANA St. C.,
Monroe 71201
Head, Dept. Biol. (B2c)

N.W. LOUISIANA St. U.,
Natchitoches 71457
Head, Dept. Biol. Sci.
(B1M2j)

LOUISIANA Polytech. Inst.,
Ruston 71270
Head, Dept. Bot. & Bact.
(B1)

LOUISIANA St. U.,
Baton Rouge 70803
Ldr., La. Coop. Wildl. Res.
Unit (BM2g)

S.W. LOUISIANA, U. of,
Lafayette 70501
WP, Dept. of Biol.
(B2j,MD3c)

MAINE, U. of, Orono 04473
Wildl. Dir., School Fr. Res.
(BMD1)S

MANITOBA, U. of,
Winnipeg, Can.
Head, Dept. Zool. (BMD3j)

MASSACHUSETTS, U. of,
Amherst 01002
Head, For. & Wildl. Dept.
(BMD1)S

McNEESE St. C.,
Lake Charles, La. 70601
WP, Agr. Dept. (B2a)

MICHIGAN, U. of,
Ann Arbor 48104
Chm., Dept. Wildl. & Fish
(BMD1)

MICHIGAN St. U.,
East Lansing 48823
Chm., Dep. Fish & Wildl.
(BMD1)

MICHIGAN Tech U.,
Houghton 49931
Head, Dept. For. (BM2g)

MINNESOTA, U. of,
St. Paul 55101
WP, Dept. Entom., Fish &
Wildl. (BMD1)

MISSISSIPPI St. U.,
State College 39762
Head, Wildl. Mgr.
(B2g,MD2j)

MISSOURI, U. of,
Columbia 65201
WP, Dept. Zool. (BMD2j)

MONTANA, U. of,
Missoula 59801
WP, School For. (BM1,D2g)S

MONTANA St. U.,
Bozeman 59715
WP, Dept. Zool. & Entom.
(BMD1)

MURRAY St. U.,
Murray, Ky. 42071
WP, Dept. Biol.-Wildl. Biol.
(BM1)

NEBRASKA, U. of,
Lincoln 68503
WP, Dept. Poultry Sci (B2a)

NEVADA, U. of, Reno 89507
WP, Renew. Res. Ctr.
(BM1)

NEW HAMPSHIRE, U. of,
Fredericton
Dir. N.E.Wildl. Sta.
(B2c,MD1)

NEW HAMPSHIRE, U. of,
Durham 03824
Dir., Inst. Nat. Environ.
Resch. (B1,M2bj)

NEW MEXICO St. U.,
Las Cruces 88001
WP, Dept. Animal, Range &
Wildl. (B2aM1)S

NEW YORK St. U.,
Syracuse 13210
Chm., Dept. For. Zool.
(BMD12jg)S

NORTH CAROLINA St. U.,
Raleigh 27607
Chm., Dept. Zool. (BMD2g)

NORTH DAKOTA U.,
Grand Forks 58202
WP, Dept. Biol.
(B1,MD2cdj)S

NORTH DAKOTA St. U.,
Fargo 58102
WP, Dept. Zool. (BMD2j)

OHIO St. U., Columbus 43210
Chm., Fac. Pop. & Envir. Biol.
(B2c,MD2j)S

OKLAHOMA St. U.,
Stillwater 74074
WP, Dept. Zool. (BMD1)

S.E. St. C. OKLAHOMA,
Durant, Okla. 74701
(B2d)

OREGON St. U.,
Corvallis 97331
Head, Dept. Fish & Wildl.
(BMD1)

PENNSYLVANIA St. U.,
University Park 16802
WP, School For. Res.
(B2g,M1,D2g)S

PURDUE U.,
Lafayette, Ind. 47907
WP, Dept. For. & Cons.
(BMD2a)

RUTGERS U.,
New Brunswick, N.J. 08903
WP, Coll. Ag. & Environ. Sci.
(B3a)

SACRAMENTO St. C.,
Sacramento, Cal. 95819
WP, Dept. Biol. Sci. (BM2c)S

SAN DIEGO St. C.,
San Diego, Cal. 92115
Chm., Dept. Biol. (BM3cdf)

SAN JOSE St. C.,
San Jose, Cal. 95114
Chm., Wildl. Cons. Curr., Biol.
Dept. (B1)

SASKATCHEWAN, U. of,
Regina and Saskatoon
WP, Dept. Biol. (BMD3c)S

SOUTH DAKOTA St. U.,
Brookings 57006
Head, Dept. Wildl. & Fish Sci.
(BM1)

TENNESSEE, U. of,
Knoxville 37916
WP, Dept. For. (BM3g)S

TENNESSEE Tech U.,
Cookeville 38501
WP, Dept. Biol. (B1,M2c)

TEXAS A & I U.,
Kingsville 78363
WP, Biol. Dept. (BM3c)

TEXAS A & M U.,
College Station 77843
WP, Dept. Wildl. Sci.
(BMD1)S

TEXAS Tech U.,
Lubbock 79409
WP, Dept. Range & Wildl.
Mgmt. (BM1,D2i)

UTAH, U. of,
Salt Lake City 84112
WP, Dept. Zool. & Ent.
(BMD3j)

UTAH St. U., Logan 84321
Head, Wildl. Res. (BMD1)S

VERMONT, U. of,
Burlington 05401
Chm., Dept. For. (B2g)

VIRGINIA Poly. Inst.,
Blacksburg 24061
WP, Dept. For. & Wildl.
(BMD1)S

WASHINGTON, U. of,
Seattle 98105
WP, Wildl. Sci., Col. For. Res.
(B1,MD3g)

WASHINGTON St. U.,
Pullman 99163
WP, Dept. Zool. (BM1,D2j)

WEST VIRGINIA U.,
Morgantown 26506
WP, Div. For. (B1,M1g)S

WISCONSIN, U. of,
Madison 53706
Chm., Dept. Wildl. Ecol.
(BMD1)

WISCONSIN St. U.,
Stevens Point 54481
WP, Dept. Nat. Res.
(B1,M2e)S

WYOMING, U. of,
Laramie 82070
Dir. Wildl. Cons., Dept. Zool.
& Phys. (BM1,D2j)S

YALE U.,
New Haven, Conn. 06520
WP, School For. (MD2dg)

MINIMUM EDUCATIONAL PROGRAM
RECOMMENDED BY THE WILDLIFE SOCIETY

The minimum educational requirements are: A full 4-year course of study in an accredited college or university leading to a bachelor's or higher degree with at least the following course requirements:

(1) 30 semester hours in biological science, which must include at least:

    (a) 6 semester hours in courses related to understanding or manipulation of environments such as principles of wildlife management, wildlife biology, environmental biology, or ecology.

    (b) 6 semester hours in vertebrate biology and classification such as mammalogy, ornithology, ichthyology or similar courses.

    (c) 9 semester hours in zoology including such subjects as general zoology, invertebrate zoology, comparative anatomy, animal physiology, genetics, parasitology or similar courses.

    (d) 9 semester hours in botany and related plant sciences in such subjects as general botany, plant taxonomy, plant ecology, or plant physiology.

(2) 15 semester hours in basic mathematics and physical science, which must include at least:

    (a) One course in college algebra or its equivalent.

    (b) One course in statistics.

    (c) One additional course each in two or more of the following: chemistry, physics, mathematics, soils, or geology.

(3) 15 semester hours in humanities and social science, which must include at least:

    (a) 4 semester hours in English composition, or demonstrated abilities (e.g. by examination) in satisfactory letter and report writing as officially certified by the university.

    (b) One course in resource economics.

RESOURCE MATERIAL ON ORGANIC GARDENING AND FARMING

From Rodale Press Book Division

SANE LIVING IN A MAD WORLD   A Guide to the Organic Way of Life

by Robert Rodale

> Sane Living in a Mad World is a basic, highly readable outline of the organic method and what it is all about. It's certain to appeal to all now involved in the organic movement and countless others who are considering this alternate life-style.
> $7.95

300 OF THE MOST ASKED QUESTIONS ABOUT ORGANIC GARDENING

Answered by the editors of Organic Gardening and Farming magazine

> Three hundred of the most-asked questions and answers on organic gardening have been assembled by experts. They tell exactly how to make compost, which insects can fight effective battles against garden pests, which fertilizers are best for lawns, vegetables and flowers, etc. All of the information is carefully organized into specific chapters then cross-referenced in a comprehensive index for easy reference.
> $6.95

WESTERN ORGANIC GARDENING

Edited by Floyd Allen

> Part I of the book relates some of the basics of organic gardening—using natural fertilizers and conditioners instead of chemicals; biological pest control methods in place of pesticides. Part II is comprised of individual gardening experiences as written for Organic Gardening and Farming by westerners who found the right methods for their unique situations.
> $6.95

THE BASIC BOOK OF ORGANICALLY GROWN FOODS

by the Editors of Organic Gardening and Farming Magazine

The book introduces the neophyte who is looking for an alternative to the over-processed, additive-laden foods sold in most stores today to a vital area of consumer concern. It reinforces the convictions and supplies additional information to those already attuned to organic foods. It's an easy reading reference book for anyone concerned about the food we eat and the world we live in.
$7.95

ORGANIC FARMING: METHODS AND MARKETS An Introduction to Ecological Agriculture

Edited by Robert Steffen, Floyd Allen and James Foote

Every day more and more ecologically-concerned farmers and would-be farmers turn to the organic way of life as the way to put an end to man's long exploitation of earth. For them, Organic Farming: Methods and Markets offers a comprehensive "bible" on all facets of farming the natural way—how to make it on a small acreage, the use of rock fertilizers, alternatives to poisonous sprays, how to produce better meat, direct-to-consumer marketing, and where to go for good advice.
$1.95 (paperback)

STEP-BY-STEP TO ORGANIC VEGETABLE GROWING

by Sam Ogden

Step-by-step illustrated instructions are included for growing more than two dozen most desired vegetables. Helpful information is given on garden planning, soil improvement, tool selection and much, much more. This is truly a standard work every organic gardener will want to read.
$6.95

THE RUTH STOUT NO-WORK GARDEN BOOK

by Ruth Stout and Richard Clemence

The book's completely tested gardening method, perfected during more than 40 years experience, eliminates gardening strain and does it organically, with no dangerous chemical fertilizers or toxic sprays.
$6.95

THE ORGANIC WAY TO MULCHING

by the editors of Organic Gardening and Farming magazine

The Organic Way to Mulching describes how to put nature's fool-proof method to work efficiently in any garden. Readers

learn how to conserve moisture, stabilize soil structure and temperature, hold down weeds and ultimately build soil fertility naturally. The book tells what mulches to use for fruits, vegetables and ornamentals and how to use them.
$5.95

THE ORGANIC WAY TO PLANT PROTECTION

by the editors of Organic Gardening and Farming magazine

The complete garden reference work on controlling insects and plant diseases naturally, without harmful pesticides. Covers vegetables, fruits, flowering plants, trees, ornamental shrubs, lawns and vines. More than 800 specific garden problems answered in over 300,000 words of down-to-earth prose. Many identifying drawings and helpful photographs. Essential reading for anyone interested in productive gardening and a safer environment.
$6.95

PAY DIRT

by J. I. Rodale

This first book on organic gardening, by the founder of the organic movement in America, is now a classic in its field. The principles set forth on soil use, nutritious food and the environment are even more meaningful today than when they were written more than 25 years ago. Pay Dirt presents the philosophy of the late Mr. Rodale, carefully developed over the years on the Organic Gardening experimental farm.
$5.95

BEST IDEAS FOR ORGANIC VEGETABLE GROWING

Compiled by the editorial staff of Organic Gardening and Farming magazine

A listing of favorite vegetables provides the procedures that successful organic gardeners have used to perform vegetable growing magic. Gardeners learn when and how to harvest without a lot of extra work, which kind of mulch works best, secrets for stretching the growing season, proper techniques for supporting and covering plants, special hints for fertilizing, which varieties do best in your area, what you can do with the space between the vegetable rows, how to beat the drought and rain, proven ways to beat bugs—and more!
$5.95

LAWN BEAUTY THE ORGANIC WAY

by the editors of Organic Gardening and Farming magazine

This concise, authoritative guide answers all the questions that annually perplex the home owner who wants a beautiful, healthy lawn. The book deals with every major insect and disease that can threaten lawns and offers safe, natural methods of control. A complete chapter discusses organic methods of weed control. $6.95

CONFESSIONS OF A SNEAKY ORGANIC COOK

by Jane Kinderlehrer

Here is the most useful guide to cooking with natural foods ever published. A rewarding book for any homemaker concerned about the possibly dangerous additives found in many of the overprocessed foods now being sold. It's a must for all those searching for new ways to provide healthy, nutritious meals— without sacrificing good taste. $6.95

From Educational Services Division of Rodale Press

INSECTS—HERE TO HELP YOU AND THE ENVIRONMENT

An 18-minute, full-color, sound filmstrip. More than 60 frames demonstrate how farmers use insects instead of DDT and other pesticides to control the pests and diseases that threaten their crops. (Includes filmstrip, cassette sound track and teacher's guide.) $13.95 (Grades 7-12)

LOOKING FOR ORGANIC AMERICA

A 27½ minute, full-color, sound filmstrip, the first in-depth study of organic farming in the United States. A visit with organic farmers from coast to coast to discover who they are and how they do it. The film makes a dramatic contrast between their creative approach and the destructive methods employed by conventional agriculture. Available for rental ($45) or purchase ($205).

COLOR ME HEALTHY

Here is a pleasant way to introduce children to basic nutritional concepts. Cartoon characters such as Hortense Honey and Rita Rye Bread tell about themselves and their nutritional value. Additional text provides basic information on vitamins, minerals, protein, proper nutritional concepts. The book may be used for simple homework assignments, as well as in the classroom. $.35 (Grades K-2)

MAKING COMPOST IN 14 DAYS

Youngsters can make their own compost piles and watch nature decompose raw organic materials into rich, natural fertilizer.

The guide for teachers and poster are designed to challenge children to undertake their own composting project, and to explain clearly how to go about it.
$1.75 (Grades 5-8)

TEACHING SCIENCE WITH GARBAGE

by Albert Schatz (professor of science education, Temple University) and Vivian Schatz (science teacher, Springside School, Philadelphia, Pa.)

This guide for teachers presents an interdisciplinary approach to environmental education. The unit will be valuable in science, mathematics and social studies classrooms. While it is ungraded, many elements of the unit will be found useful from lower elementary grades through junior high school.

The emphasis in this unit is on composting or microbial decomposition under controlled conditions. Simple experiments demonstrate the changes that garbage undergoes. It's important to note that the materials needed for the experiments are simple, inexpensive, readily available and familiar (garbage, soil, nails, steel wool, etc.)
$1.50, 60 pages—illustrated with drawings, photographs and charts. Biblio. (Paperback)

THE ORGANIC CLASSROOM   An Introduction to Environmental Education—The Organic Way

Planned for use throughout the school year, the Organic Classroom includes more than 30 suggested interdisciplinary activities and projects. Some examples:

Make your own breakfast cereal (a simple recipe to teach youngsters the difference between "empty" and nutritious calories).

Grow an herb garden (to acquaint youngsters with the variety of seasonings available in addition to salt and pepper).

Walk like an animal (an on-going exercise routine to condition and loosen muscles).

Build soil (to teach the components of soil—particularly the organic material).

Sprout seeds (to demonstrate how environmental factors affect plant growth).

Raise worms (they aerate and fertilize the soil—easy to see in a glass tank).

Recycle your garbage (the classroom can be a miniature recycling plant, a practical solution to solid waste pollution).
$1.50 (Grades K-8)

ENCYCLOPEDIA OF ORGANIC GARDENING

by J. I. Rodale and Staff

Here is the complete how-to-do-it of organic gardening from A to Z, written in easy-to-understand, nontechnical language. Here are some of the hundreds of subjects covered: flower garden, vegetable garden, soils, fruits and nuts, composting, homesteading, and greenhouse gardening.
$11.95

INDEX

207